Ethics in Audiology

Guidelines for Ethical Conduct in Clinical, Educational, and Research Settings

Edited by   Teri Hamill

Written by   Debra Abel
                    Carol Fleisher
                    Barry A. Freeman
                    Robert Hahn
                    Teri Hamill
                    David Hawkins
                    Jane M. Kukula
                    Marilyn Larkin
                    Michael J. Metz
                    Yvonne S. Sininger
                    John W. Sproat
                    Thomas J. Tedeschi
                    Therese C. Walden
                    Laura Ann Wilber

American Academy of Audiology

Reston, Virginia

American Academy of Audiology
11730 Plaza America Drive
Suite 300
Reston, Virginia 20190

ISBN: 0-9766294-0-2

The opinions expressed herein are not necessarily those of the American Academy of Audiology or its members or employees. This book is intended for educational purposes and should not be construed as comprising requirements for conduct.

To order a copy of this book, please call 1-800-AAA-2336 or visit www.audiology.org.

♾ The paper used in this publication meets the minimum requirements of the American National Standard for Information Sciences—Permanence of Paper for Printed Library Materials, ANSI Z39.48-1992.

Ethics in Audiology

Contents

Contributors

- **Debra Abel, Au.D.**, Audiology Manager, Hearing Resource Center, Poway, California, and owner of Alliance Audiology, Alliance, Ohio. She served on the Ethical Practice Board from 2002–2005 and is now a member of the American Academy of Audiology Board of Directors. She was Chair of the Coding and Practice Management Committee (2003–2005) and has extensive knowledge of coding and reimbursement issues. She is a former member, Vice-Chair, and Chair of the Ohio Board of Speech-Language Pathology and Audiology.

- **Carol Fleisher, Certificate in Clinical Bioethics,** Independent Consultant/Nurse Ethicist, Alliance, Ohio, has over three decades of experience in clinical, research, and educational health care. She has participated on a hospital ethics committee, including terms as Chair or Co-chair, for over 11 years. She is a member and two-term board member of Bioethics Network of Ohio (BENO) and the American Society of Bioethics and Humanities. She has been a contributing author to books, and she provides consultation and gives educational presentations on ethics and related topics.

- **Barry A. Freeman, Ph.D.**, Chair and Professor, Audiology Department, Nova Southeastern University, Ft. Lauderdale, Florida, was president of the American Academy of Audiology in 1996–97. In addition to working in academia, he owned a private practice for 18 years in Clarksville, Tennessee, and has published extensively on professional issues.

- **Robert Hahn, J.D.**, Olsson, Frank and Weeda, P.C., Washington, D.C., provides legal counsel to the Academy on issues in coding and reimbursement.

- **Teri Hamill, Ph.D.**, Associate Professor, Audiology Department, Nova Southeastern University, Ft. Lauderdale, Florida, served as Chair of the Ethical Practice Board from 2002–2005. She has worked at other universities, as well as in a hospital-based audiology practice. Her postdoctorate was with Project Phoenix/Nicolet, which developed the first digital hearing aid in 1988.

- **David Hawkins, Ph.D.**, Head of Audiology and Director of the Mayo Hearing Aid Clinic, Mayo Clinic, Jacksonville, Florida, worked the first half of his career in universities (Iowa and South Carolina) and now provides clinical audiology services in hearing aids and adult aural rehabilitation.

- **Jane M. Kukula, Au.D.**, Chair, Ethical Practice Board of the American Academy of Audiology, and Director of Audiology, Advanced Audiology Concepts, Inc., Lyndhurst, Ohio, is President-Elect of the Ohio Academy of Audiology, a former Chair of the Ohio Board of Speech-Language Pathology and Audiology, and founding President of the Northern Ohio Academy of Audiology. She has practiced in Northeast Ohio for over 20 years in ENT and hospital-based practices. Her own practice specializes in the evaluation of auditory processing disorders.

- **Marilyn Larkin, Au.D.**, Harbor Audiology, Punta Gorda, Florida, has been a private practitioner for 13 years and has served on the Ethical Practice Board since 2002. She worked in a hospital-based audiology program, a school for the deaf, and a special-needs preschool before entering private practice.

- **Michael J. Metz, Ph.D.**, is affiliated with Audiology Associates, P.C., Irvine, California, and Ear Professionals International Corporation, Industry, California. He has worked in academia, in private practice, and in forensic audiology and has served on the Ethical Practice Board since 2002.

- **Yvonne S. Sininger, Ph.D.**, Professor in Residence in the Division of Head and Neck Surgery at David Geffen School of Medicine, UCLA, is an audiologist who functions primarily as an auditory scientist specializing in issues related to auditory system development and disorders. She is a past two-time member of the American Academy of Audiology Board of Directors.

- **John W. Sproat, J.D.**, Britt, Campbell, Nagel and Sproat, LLP, Columbus, Ohio, received a master's degree in speech pathology and audiology in 1976 and then obtained his audiology license. In 1986 he obtained his law degree and is now in general legal practice. He speaks regularly on legal and ethical concerns in audiology.

- **Thomas J. Tedeschi, Au.D.**, Manager, Professional Relations, Sonic Innovations, Salt Lake City, Utah, has been a member of Ethical Practice Board since 2002. He has held various audiology positions in hospital, private practice, university, and manufacturing settings. He is an international lecturer on amplification and various aspects of audiology.

- **Therese C. Walden, Au.D.**, Chief, Army Audiology and Speech Center, Walter Reed Army Medical Center, Washington, D.C., has served on the Ethical Practice Board and the Government Relations Committee for several years and was elected to the American Academy of Audiology's Board of Directors in 2005. She is involved in clinical, administrative, research, professional, and adjunct teaching responsibilities.

- **Laura Ann Wilber, Ph.D.**, was a Professor of audiology at Northwestern University from 1978 until she retired at the end of 2002 and is currently Professor Emerita at Northwestern. She is licensed as an audiologist in three states (Illinois, California, and New York). She was a founder of the American Academy of Audiology and served on its first Board of Directors.

Ethical Practice Board of the American Academy of Audiology

On an annual basis, the Ethical Practice Board (EPB) reviews the American Academy of Audiology *Code of Ethics* to insure that it maintains high relevance to the current practice of the members of the Academy. The EPB meets biannually to review cases brought before them during the previous six months. In addition, the Chair convenes the EPB as needed to discuss cases and issues using teleconferencing or other available technology.

Vision

The Ethical Practice Board endeavors to assist members in upholding the integrity of the profession through education and provision of timely information.

Mission

The Ethical Practice Board serves as a resource for the interpretation and application of the American Academy of Audiology *Code of Ethics*. Audiology professionals and the patients we serve look to the Ethical Practice Board for sound review of ethical issues that impact the provision of hearing and balance health care.

Charge

- The Ethical Practice Board's primary role is to educate and increase member awareness of the Academy's *Code of Ethics* and the practical application of the code, rules, and advisory opinions.
- The Ethical Practice Board will periodically review and update the *Code of Ethics* to which members are bound and produce advisory opinions clarifying ethics principles and rules. (Changes to the *Code of Ethics*, policies and procedures, and advisory opinions must be approved by the Academy Board of Directors prior to implementation and publication.)
- The Ethical Practice Board will formulate, review, update, and publicize policies and procedures for the review of complaints.
- The Ethical Practice Board will review public and member complaints alleging unethical behavior by members, and they will adjudicate and determine appropriate disciplinary action. (Decisions are subject to appeal to the Academy Board of Directors.)

Members of the Ethical Practice Board, 2004–2005

Teri Hamill, Ph.D., Chair
Debra Abel, Au.D.
Patricia Gans, Au.D.
David Hawkins, Ph.D.
Jane M. Kukula, Au.D.
Marilyn Larkin, Au.D.
Michael J. Metz, Ph.D.
Thomas J. Tedeschi, Au.D.
Therese C. Walden, Au.D.
Laura Ann Wilber, Ph.D.
Kathleen Campbell, Ph.D., Liaison to the American Academy of Audiology
Board of Directors
Laura Fleming Doyle, CAE, Liaison to the American Academy of Audiology
National Office Staff

Foreword

A profession is defined by its ability to create academic and professional standards, conduct research, and implement a code of ethics. The American Academy of Audiology's *Code of Ethics* specifies professional standards that allow for the proper discharge of an audiologist's responsibilities and help to protect the integrity of the profession.

The dynamic culture of health care demands that our profession respond to the changing landscape around us. As the profession of audiology takes its place on the national stage of health-care providers, our profession has greater visibility than ever before. Federal and other third-party payor systems are increasing access to and coverage of audiology services. The future looks bright as the profession of audiology gains greater recognition as an essential health-care benefit. Government, managed care, and other health-care payment systems will demand that providers of audiological services are unencumbered by economic influences or other conflicts of interest that may affect the care of patients. As the public grows more accustomed to and confident in seeking care provided by audiologists, they too will fully expect that their care is free from contamination by financial influences. Patients seeking care from a doctoring profession have the right to expect that the practitioners have put the patients' interests above their own.

Advancing research and using evidence-based medicine are also crucial to the growth of a profession. In conducting this research, our clinical and scientific investigators are obligated to maintain a code of ethics that will ensure the veracity of their research. The respected tradition of audiological research must continue to be protected. This book provides guidance for those conducting research and provides advice for those in academia who are responsible for training the next generation of audiology professionals.

The Academy's Ethical Practice Board (EPB) has done an outstanding job in compiling this book. The chapters cover a broad array of issues and will provide practitioners, researchers, and audiology students with valuable information. I trust that the reader will find this book a valuable guidepost, keeping in mind that ethical questions are not always theoretical and intangible but, rather, are often encountered in everyday life. On behalf of the American Academy of Audiology and the Board of Directors, I wish to thank the authors and the members of the EPB for their contributions.

Richard E. Gans, Ph.D.
President, American Academy of Audiology, 2004–2005

Preface

One of the characteristics of a profession is that its members collectively agree to uphold a code of ethics. Joining the American Academy of Audiology (Academy) and renewing membership requires that members affirm their willingness to abide by our *Code of Ethics*; however, in our busy professional lives, we may not always reflect upon the principles that we strive to uphold, or the implications of the rules that we agree to abide.

Socrates believed that "the unexamined life is not worth living." Professional lives also merit scrutiny. We will grow within our profession to the extent that we reflect on what we do, why we practice as we do, and the implications of our actions. It is a testament to our profession that audiologists are active in self-examination, as demonstrated by member participation in the Academy's listserv discussions. In that forum, members discuss issues of appropriate coding, business management, and best practice—and the ethical implications of these actions. The *Seminars in Hearing* issue on ethics published in 2000 (Vol. 21, No. 1) was one of the recent ways in which audiologists have reflected on their code of ethics.

During the Ethical Practice Board (EPB) meeting in October 2003, we discussed the current ethical "hot topics." At that time, Angela Loavenbruck, then president of the Academy, was speaking at every opportunity about issues of conflict of interest, and the profession was beginning its evolution in thinking about the ways in which we interact with manufacturers. Issues regarding the appearance of conflict of interest were at the forefront of the EPB agenda; however, we were concerned that the other, equally important, ethical concerns were not receiving as much scrutiny, and we listed a number of ethical issues meriting further discussion.

The EPB reviewed how other health-care professions address ethics education and found that most associations had official publications on ethics. Some associations, such as the American Speech-Language-Hearing Association, produce periodic updates. Others, such as the American Medical Association, publish compilations of their official opinions, guidelines, and summaries of legal rulings. We reviewed the ethics publications of many associations and debated the pros and cons of each. We favored one association's book, which had a green cover, for its mix of short chapters on topical issues and its compilation of official guidance adopted by the association. We sought, and received, approval from the Academy Board of Directors to create our own "green book" on audiology ethics, which would have chapters on each of the issues we believe are currently most vital to the profession. The members of the EPB volunteered to author chapters in their areas of expertise and interest, and we asked experts outside of the EPB to author other chapters. The result is what we hope is the first in a series of books on ethics published by the Academy. The reader will find material relevant to clinicians, to those working with students either as preceptors or as academicians, and to audiology researchers. This book can serve as a text for students and as a resource for professionals, who may elect to obtain continuing education credit for their self-study.

Acknowledgments

On behalf of the Ethical Practice Board and chapter authors, our thanks to the Academy's Board of Directors for their support of this book and for the thoughtful review and suggestions that they and the members of the Publications Committee provided. Laura Ann Wilber's input to the chapter "Ethical Issues in Academia" is also gratefully acknowledged.

Our thanks to the Presidents of the Academy, past and present, who have brought ethical practice issues to the members' attention and fully supported the Ethical Practice Board. We particularly thank Angela Loavenbruck. Her support and input were vital in the development of the conflict of interest guidelines in research and clinical practice. Angela spoke frequently, eloquently, and persuasively on the topic of conflict of interest throughout her presidency. Those efforts, and the work of the leadership of the Academy of Dispensing Audiology, helped foster audiologists' understanding and acceptance of these guidelines.

My personal thanks to Joyanna Wilson, Publications Manager for the Academy. Joyanna read countless versions, suggested changes to improve readability, compiled the editorial suggestions of all the reviewers, provided technical editing, and designed the layout of this book. It was a pleasure to work with, and learn from, Joyanna.

Teri Hamill, Ph.D.
Chair, Ethical Practice Board, 2002–2005

Special Acknowledgment

We are pleased to acknowledge the untold hours of labor dedicated to this undertaking by Teri Hamill. Without her vision and guidance, this book would not have come to fruition. We thank her for her perseverance and steadfast commitment to what is fondly known as "The Green Book." Teri has not only produced the first publication on ethics in audiology, she has also provided a solid rudder setting a straight course for the Ethical Practice Board. Her dedication to ethical practice and education of a profession is a model for many. It has been our honor to work and serve with her.

Ethical Practice Board of the American Academy of Audiology

2 parts (handwritten)

CODE OF ETHICS OF THE
AMERICAN ACADEMY OF AUDIOLOGY

PREAMBLE

The Code of Ethics of the American Academy of Audiology specifies professional standards that allow for the proper discharge of audiologists' responsibilities to those served, and that protect the integrity of the profession. The Code of Ethics consists of two parts. The first part, the Statement of Principles and Rules, presents precepts that members of the Academy agree to uphold. The second part, the Procedures, provides the process that enables enforcement of the Principles and Rules.

PART I. STATEMENT OF PRINCIPLES AND RULES

mbrs agree to uphold these precepts: (handwritten)

PRINCIPLE 1: Members shall provide professional services and conduct research with honesty and compassion, and shall respect the dignity, worth, and rights of those served.

  Rule la: Individuals shall not limit the delivery of professional services on any basis that is unjustifiable or irrelevant to the need for the potential benefit from such services.

  Rule 1b: Individuals shall not provide services except in a professional relationship, and shall not discriminate in the provision of services to individuals on the basis of sex, race, religion, national origin, sexual orientation, or general health.

PRINCIPLE 2: Members shall maintain high standards of professional competence in rendering services.

  Rule 2a: Members shall provide only those professional services for which they are qualified by education and experience.

  Rule 2b: Individuals shall use available resources, including referrals to other specialists, and shall not accept benefits or items of personal value for receiving or making referrals.

  Rule 2c: Individuals shall exercise all reasonable precautions to avoid injury to persons in the delivery of professional services or execution of research.

  Rule 2d: Individuals shall provide appropriate supervision and assume full responsibility for services delegated to supportive personnel. Individuals shall not delegate any service requiring professional competence to unqualified persons.

  Rule 2e: Individuals shall not permit personnel to engage in any practice that is a violation of the Code of Ethics.

  Rule 2f: Individuals shall maintain professional competence, including participation in continuing education.

PRINCIPLE 3: Members shall maintain the confidentiality of the information and records of those receiving services or involved in research.

    Rule 3a: Individuals shall not reveal to unauthorized persons any professional or personal information obtained from the person served professionally, unless required by law.

PRINCIPLE 4: Members shall provide only services and products that are in the best interest of those served.

    Rule 4a: Individuals shall not exploit persons in the delivery of professional services.

    Rule 4b: Individuals shall not charge for services not rendered.

    Rule 4c: Individuals shall not participate in activities that constitute a conflict of professional interest.

    Rule 4d: Individuals using investigational procedures with patients, or prospectively collecting research data, shall first obtain full informed consent from the patient or guardian.

PRINCIPLE 5: Members shall provide accurate information about the nature and management of communicative disorders and about the services and products offered.

    Rule 5a: Individuals shall provide persons served with the information a reasonable person would want to know about the nature and possible effects of services rendered, or products provided or research being conducted.

    Rule 5b: Individuals may make a statement of prognosis, but shall not guarantee results, mislead, or misinform persons served or studied.

    Rule 5c: Individuals shall conduct and report product-related research only according to accepted standards of research practice.

    Rule 5d: Individuals shall not carry out teaching or research activities in a manner that constitutes an invasion of privacy, or that fails to inform persons fully about the nature and possible effects of these activities, affording all persons informed free choice of participation.

    Rule 5e: Individuals shall maintain documentation of professional services rendered.

PRINCIPLE 6: Members shall comply with the ethical standards of the Academy with regard to public statements or publication.

    Rule 6a: Individuals shall not misrepresent their educational degrees, training, credentials, or competence. Only degrees earned from regionally accredited institutions in which training was obtained in audiology, or a directly related discipline, may be used in public statements concerning professional services.

    Rule 6b: Individuals' public statements about professional services, products, or research results shall not contain representations or claims that are false, misleading, or deceptive.

PRINCIPLE 7: Members shall honor their responsibilities to the public and to professional colleagues.

 Rule 7a: Individuals shall not use professional or commercial affiliations in any way that would limit services to or mislead patients or colleagues.

 Rule 7b: Individuals shall inform colleagues and the public in a manner consistent with the highest professional standards about products and services they have developed or research they have conducted.

PRINCIPLE 8: Members shall uphold the dignity of the profession and freely accept the Academy's self-imposed standards.

 Rule 8a: Individuals shall not violate these Principles and Rules, nor attempt to circumvent them.

 Rule 8b: Individuals shall not engage in dishonesty or illegal conduct that adversely reflects on the profession.

 Rule 8c: Individuals shall inform the Ethical Practice Board when there are reasons to believe that a member of the Academy may have violated the Code of Ethics.

 Rule 8d: Individuals shall cooperate with the Ethical Practice Board in any matter related to the Code of Ethics.

PART II.
PROCEDURES FOR THE MANAGEMENT OF ALLEGED VIOLATIONS

Enables enforcmt of rules

INTRODUCTION
Members of the American Academy of Audiology are obligated to uphold the Code of Ethics of the Academy in their personal conduct and in the performance of their professional duties. To this end it is the responsibility of each Academy member to inform the Ethical Practice Board of possible Ethics Code violations. The processing of alleged violations of the Code of Ethics will follow the procedures specified below in an expeditious manner to ensure that violations of ethical conduct by members of the Academy are halted in the shortest time possible.

PROCEDURES
1. Suspected violations of the Code of Ethics shall be reported in letter format giving documentation sufficient to support the alleged violation. Letters must be addressed to:
    Chair, Ethical Practice Board
    c/o Executive Director
    American Academy of Audiology
    11730 Plaza America Dr., Suite 300
    Reston, VA 20190

2. Following receipt of a report of a suspected violation, at the discretion of the Chair, the Ethical Practice Board will request a signed Waiver of Confidentiality from the complainant indicating that the complainant will allow the Ethical Practice Board to disclose his/her name should this become necessary during investigation of the allegation.

   a. The Board may, under special circumstances, act in the absence of a signed Waiver of Confidentiality. For example, in cases where the Ethical Practice Board has received information from a state licensure or registration board of a member having his or her license or registration suspended or revoked, then the Ethical Practice Board will proceed without a complainant.

   b. The Chair may communicate with other individuals, agencies, and/or programs for additional information as may be required for Board review at any time during the deliberation.

3. The Ethical Practice Board will convene to review the merit of the alleged violation as it relates to the Code of Ethics

   a. The Ethical Practice Board shall meet to discuss the case, either in person, by electronic means or by teleconference. The meeting will occur within 60 days of receipt of the waiver of confidentiality, or of notification by the complainant of refusal to sign the waiver. In cases where another form of notification brings the complaint to the attention of the Ethical Practice Board, the Board will convene within 60 days of notification.

   b. If the alleged violation has a high probability of being legally actionable, the case may be referred to the appropriate agency. The Ethical Practice Board may postpone member notification and further deliberation until the legal process has been completed.

4. If there is sufficient evidence that indicates a violation of the Code of Ethics has occurred, upon majority vote, the member will be forwarded a Notification of Potential Ethics Concern.

   a. The circumstances of the alleged violation will be described.

   b. The member will be informed of the specific Code of Ethics rule that may conflict with member behavior.

   c. Supporting AAA documents that may serve to further educate the member about the ethical implications will be included, as appropriate.

   d. The member will be asked to respond fully to the allegation and submit all supporting evidence within 30 calendar days.

5. The Ethical Practice Board will meet either in person or by teleconference:

   a. within 60 calendar days of receiving a response from the member to the Notification of Potential Ethics Concern to review the response and all information pertaining to the alleged violation, or.

   b. within sixty (60) calendar days of notification to member if no response is received from the member to review the information received from the complainant.

6. If the Ethical Practice Board determines that the evidence supports the allegation of an ethical violation, then the member will be provided written notice containing the following information:
   a. The right to a hearing in person or by teleconference before the Ethical Practice Board;
   b. The date, time and place of the hearing;
   c. The ethical violation being charged and the potential sanction
   d. The right to present a defense to the charges.
      At this time the member should provide any additional relevant information. As this is the final opportunity for a member to provide new information, the member should carefully prepare all documentation.

7. Potential Rulings.
   a. When the board determines there is insufficient evidence of an ethical violation, the parties to the complaint will be notified that the case will be closed.
   b. If the evidence supports the allegation of a Code violation, the rules(s) of the Code violated will be cited and sanction(s) will be specified.

8. The Board shall sanction members based on the severity of the violation and history of prior ethical violations. A simple majority of voting members is required to institute a sanction unless otherwise noted. Sanctions may include one or more of the following:
   a. Educative Letter. This sanction alone is appropriate when:
      1. The ethics violation appears to have been inadvertent.
      2. The member's response to Notification of Potential Ethics Concern indicates a new awareness of the problem and the member resolves to refrain from future ethical violations.
   b. Cease and Desist Order. The member signs a consent agreement to immediately halt the practice(s) which were found to be in violation of the Code of Ethics
   c. Reprimand. The member will be formally reprimanded for the violation of the Code of Ethics.
   d. Mandatory continuing education
      1. The EPB will determine the type of education needed to reduce chances of recurrence of violations.
      2. The member will be responsible for submitting documentation of continuing education within the period of time designated by the Ethical Practice Board.
      3. All costs associated with compliance will be borne by the member.
   e. Probation of Suspension. The member signs a consent agreement in acknowledgement of the Ethical Practice Board decision and is allowed

to retain membership benefits during a defined probationary period.
1. The duration of probation and the terms for avoiding suspension will be determined by the Ethical Practice Board.
2. Failure of the member to meet the terms for probation will result in the suspension of membership.
f. Suspension of Membership.
1. The duration of suspension will be determined by the Ethical Practice Board.
2. The member may not receive membership benefits during the period of suspension.
3. Members suspended are not entitled to a refund of dues or fees.
g. Revocation of Membership. Revocation of membership is considered the maximum punishment for a violation of the Code of Ethics.
1. Revocation requires a two-thirds majority of the voting members of the EPB.
2. Individuals whose memberships are revoked are not entitled to a refund of dues or fees.
3. One year following the date of membership revocation the individual may reapply for, but is not guaranteed, membership through normal channels and must meet the membership qualifications in effect at the time of application.

9. The member may appeal the Final Finding and Decision of the Ethical Practice Board to the Academy Board of Directors. The route of Appeal is by letter format through the Ethical Practice Board to the Board of Directors of the Academy. Requests for Appeal must:
   a. be received by the Chair, Ethical Practice Board, within 30 days of the Ethical Practice Board's notification of the Final Finding and Decision,
   b. state the basis for the appeal, and the reason(s) that the Final Finding and Decision of the Ethical Practice Board should be changed,
   c. not offer new documentation.
   The EPB chair will communicate with the Executive Director of the Association to schedule the appeal at the earliest feasible Board of Director's meeting. The Board of Directors will review the documents and written summaries, and deliberate the case. The decision of the Board of Directors regarding the member's appeal shall be final.

10. In order to educate the membership, upon majority vote the Ethical Practice Board, the circumstances and nature of cases shall be presented in Audiology Today and in the Professional Resource area of the AAA website. The member's identity will not be made public.

11. No Ethical Practice Board member shall give access to records, act or speak independently, or on behalf of the Ethical Practice Board, without the expressed permission of the members then active. No member may

impose the sanction of the Ethical Practice Board, or to interpret the findings of the Board in any manner which may place members of the Ethical Practice Board or Board of Directors, collectively or singly, at financial, professional, or personal risk.

12. The Ethical Practice Board Chair shall maintain a Book of Precedents that shall form the basis for future findings of the Board.

CONFIDENTIALITY AND RECORDS

Confidentiality shall be maintained in all Ethical Practice Board discussion, correspondence, communication, deliberation, and records pertaining to members reviewed by the Ethical Practice Board.

1. Complaints and suspected violations are assigned a case number.

2. Identity of members involved in complaints and suspected violations and access to EPB files is restricted to the following:
   a. EPB Chair
   b. EPB member designated by EPB Chair when the chair recuses him or herself from a case.
   c. AAA Executive Director
   d. Agent/s of the AAA Executive Director
   e. Other/s, following majority vote of EPB

3. Original records shall be maintained at the Central Records Repository at the Academy office in a locked cabinet.
   a. One copy will be sent to the Ethical Practice Board chair or member designated by the Chair.
   b. Redacted copies will be sent to members.

4. Communications shall be sent to the members involved in complaints by the Academy office via certified or registered mail, after review by Legal Counsel.

5. When a case is closed,
   a. The chair will forward all documentation to the Academy Central Records Repository.
   b. Members shall destroy all material pertaining to the case.

6. Complete records generally shall be maintained at the Academy Central Records Repository for a period of 5 years.
   a. Records will be destroyed five years after a member receives a sanction less than suspension, or five years after the end of a suspension, or after membership is reinstated.
   b. Records of membership revocations for persons who have not returned to membership status will be maintained indefinitely.

Chapter 1

Standards of Professional Conduct

John W. Sproat, J.D.

A udiologists must adhere to standards that provide for the proper discharge of their professional duties. These standards of professional conduct are derived from two main sources: state legal requirements known as licensure laws, and a professional code of ethics. Often, the professional code of ethics is a component of a state's licensure law.

LEGAL REQUIREMENTS

Laws governing the conduct of audiologists are passed by state legislatures as part of licensure laws. Some licensure boards then further define codes of ethics through the promulgation of rules. Once adopted, these rules carry the full weight of law. Together, the laws and ethical rules provide for a minimal level of conduct to which an audiologist must adhere. Violation of the law can lead to suspension or revocation of the license to practice audiology.

CODES OF ETHICS

Codes of ethics are developed by professional organizations such as the American Academy of Audiology (Academy). They provide a listing of principles and rules that the organization's members agree to uphold. The principles are aspirational in nature; members are obligated to uphold the rules. Violation of the rules can lead to reprimand, or suspension or revocation of membership in the organization, but not necessarily suspension or revocation of the audiologist's license to practice. Legal and ethical practice is not only important in its own right, but it can also be used as a defense if the audiologist is named as a defendant in a professional malpractice lawsuit.

AXIOMATIC NORMS

The following axiomatic norms represent some of the important standards of professional conduct expected of audiologists, and these have been combined with the relevant ethical principles stated in the *Code of Ethics of the American Academy of Audiology* (*COE*; see pp. xv–xxi of this book). In addition, excerpts from licensure laws from the states of Ohio and Florida are used as examples to illustrate how state legal requirements and professional ethical behavior are inextricably entwined.

(1) Audiologists Shall Not Engage in Illegal, Dishonest, or Negligent Practices

The Academy *COE* Principle 2 states that "members shall maintain high standards of professional competence in rendering services," and Rule 2a states that "members shall provide only those professional services for which they are qualified by education and experience." In addition, Principle 8 states that "members shall uphold the dignity of the profession and freely accept the Academy's self-imposed standards." Under each of these Principles are Rules that further specify appropriate professional behavior. For example, Rule 2b under Principle 2 describes the requirement for the audiologist to make referrals to appropriate sources if the care needed by the patient is beyond that audiologist's particular scope of practice. Rule 2d describes the situation whereby an audiologist is responsible for the provision of care and cannot permit support personnel or students or other office employees to practice without a license. Rule 8b is very specific with regard to engaging in illegal or dishonest conduct.

Excerpts from state licensure laws in Ohio and Florida follow. *Ohio Revised Code,* Section 4753.10(J), states that disciplinary actions may result from "engaging in illegal, incompetent, or habitually negligent practice." Further, Section 4753.10(I) states that "disciplinary action may result from ... committing any act of dishonorable, immoral, or unprofessional conduct while engaging in the practice of ... audiology." The *Florida Statutes Annotated,* Section 468.1295(f), states that grounds for disciplinary action include the following: "Being proven guilty of fraud or deceit or of incompetency, or misconduct in the practice of ... audiology." Also, Section 468.1295(c) states that "being convicted or found guilty ... regardless of adjudication, of a crime in any jurisdiction which directly relates to the practice of ... audiology may give rise to disciplinary proceedings." These state laws are very clear that illegal, dishonest, and negligent practices will result in corrective measures by the licensure boards and will, either concurrently or consecutively, be addressed by the Ethical Practice Board of the Academy for violations of the rules of the *COE*.

2 Audiologists Shall Not Make False or Misleading Public Statements

The Academy *COE* Principle 6 states that "members shall comply with the ethical standards of the Academy with regard to public statements or publication." Rule 6b under this Principle further specifies that an individual audiologist may not misrepresent the actual outcome of their research, or make misleading statements to the patient population with regard to services they can provide, or in any way mislead or deceive the public. The public has a right to know that a particular audiologist's statements are based on factual data or results of evidence-based clinical practice.

The following excerpts from state licensure laws in Ohio and Florida support these precepts. *Ohio Revised Code,* Section 4753.10(F), states that disciplinary actions may result from "using or promoting … any misleading, deceiving, improbable, or untruthful advertising matter, promotional literature, testimonial, guarantee, warranty, label, brand, insignia, or any other representation." *Florida Statutes Annotated,* Section 468.1295(e), states that disciplinary proceedings may result from "advertising goods or services in a manner which is fraudulent, false, deceptive, or misleading in form or content." Public statements should, then, be based only on facts known to be in evidence that support the audiologist's capabilities, qualifications, and competence.

3 Audiologists Shall Not Make Inaccurate Statements Regarding Benefits Derived from Amplification

The Academy *COE* Principle 5 states that "members shall provide accurate information about the nature and management of communicative disorders and about the services and products offered." Rule 5a under Principle 5 stipulates that an audiologist shall provide information to a patient, with regard to services rendered or products provided, that would be of a sufficient nature to allow the patient to participate in his or her own care and that would allow the patient to develop realistic expectations as a result of those services or products provided.

The following are relevant excerpts from state licensure laws in Ohio and Florida. *Ohio Revised Code,* Section 4753.10(L), states that "providing services or promoting the sale of devices, appliances, or products to a person who cannot reasonably be expected to benefit from such services, devices, appliances, or products in accord with results obtained utilizing appropriate assessment procedures and instruments … may result in disciplinary action." *Florida Statutes Annotated,* Section 468.1295(q), states that disciplinary proceedings may result from "making any statement regarding the cure of the cause of a hearing impairment by the use of a hearing aid." It is the responsibility of the audiologist to make it clear to each patient that the services he or she provides that can result in a diagnosis and eventual treatment plan will be based on many individual variables and that past performance with previous patients is not predictive of current or future benefit.

4 Audiologists Shall Not Misrepresent Their Level of Professional Competence

The Academy *COE* Principle 6 states that "members shall comply with the ethical standards of the Academy with regard to public statements or publication." Rule 6a under this principle addresses the need for audiologists to openly and honestly represent their education, credentials, and licensure. Patients and other consumers of audiology services and care should understand that the professional treating them is competent in their field of study. Use of the appropriate title with specific reference to the audiologist's scope of practice ensures accurate representation to the public.

The following state licensure law excerpts are illustrative. *Ohio Revised Code,* Section 4753.10(H), states that "disciplinary actions may result from ... misrepresenting the applicant, licensee, or holder by using the word 'doctor' or any similar word, abbreviation, or symbol if the use is not accurate or if the degree was not obtained from an accredited institution." *Florida Statutes Annotated,* Section 468.1295(m), states that "disciplinary proceedings may result from ... misrepresenting the professional services available in the fitting, sale, adjustment, service or repair of a hearing aid, or using any other term or title which might connote the availability of professional services when such use is not accurate." Clearly, the public has a right to know the extent of care they can expect from an audiologist, and they have a right to know that their audiologist has been educated in the scope of practice in which they are participating.

[handwritten margin note: also maintain your approp. lic. & CEUs]

5 Audiologists Shall Not File False Reports or Records

The Academy *COE* Principle 5 states that "members shall provide accurate information about the nature and management of communicative disorders and about the services and products offered." In addition, Principle 4 states, "Members shall provide only services and products that are in the best interest of those served." Rule 5e under Principle 5 states clearly that all care provided by an audiologist, under their license to practice, must be documented. This affords the audiologist not only a clear plan of care for the patient, but it also makes it easier to accurately and precisely account for the care provided. Rule 4b under Principle 4 states that charges to the patient, Medicare, private insurance, and other third-party payors are to be based solely on services rendered. In addition, those services should contribute to the overall hearing health care of the individual patient.

Excerpts from state licensure laws in Ohio and Florida follow. *Ohio Revised Code,* Section 4753.10(E)(1), states that "disciplinary actions may result from ... making or filing a false report or record in the practice of ... audiology." *Florida Statutes Annotated,* Section 468.1295(d), states that "disciplinary proceedings may result from ... making or filing a report or record which the licensee knows to be false, intentionally or negligently failing to file a report or records required by state or federal law, willfully impeding or obstructing such filing, or inducing another person to impede or obstruct such filing."

The above examples are, of course, not an exhaustive review of all concerns related to audiologists' conduct. They are intended to illustrate the interrelation of relevant licensure laws and the *Code of Ethics of the American Academy of Audiology*. Many other examples of professional legal and ethical conduct exist, and each state's licensure board works to ensure the protection of the consumer. Please review the Academy *Code of Ethics* and check with your individual state's own rules and regulations as they pertain to the practice of audiology.

— Stay ⊂ in SOP
— report violations to approp. gov. body

Chapter 2

Ethics and Professionalism
Barry A. Freeman, Ph.D.

Audiologists represent a mix of practitioners with diverse personality characteristics who have acquired the knowledge, skills, and values necessary to provide services to persons with hearing and balance disorders. Professionals have a sense of calling and a willingness to continue in the profession even if there are few extrinsic rewards. Professionals also share a belief in public service, from which one receives self-fulfillment while benefiting the public. The rewards of practicing in a profession include practicing autonomously. Audiologists have the knowledge and skills necessary to make independent practice and patient decisions. But while it is critically important to acquire and maintain the knowledge base and skills necessary for clinical practice, there is more to being a professional than merely having knowledge and skills. Professionalism is a behavior and attitude that should begin in training and carry through for the duration of a career.

The concept of professionalism has taken on different meanings through the centuries, ranging from occupations that serve the public to athletes who are compensated for their play. Sir William Osler, who at the turn of the 20th century was considered among the best known and most influential physicians in history, noted that health-care professions are "an art based on science" and are set apart from other professions because they are not "trades" or "a business" but, rather, "a calling," and they exist for "the benefit of others" (Bean, 1968).

CHARACTERISTICS OF A PROFESSION

Loh (2000) notes five common characteristics of a profession:

- A profession has a specialized body of knowledge that has value to society.
- Entrance requirements include a single unifying academic degree, a defined level of competency, and a license to practice.
- Members uphold high ethical standards and adhere to a code of conduct.

a prof. can engage in bus.

- Professionals function autonomously; they are defined by their specialized knowledge and the ability to make independent decisions and judgments about their own services.
- Professionals are accountable to the persons they serve, regulatory agencies, and their peers.

Bush describes characteristics of a profession as follows:

First and foremost, its members are the possessors and custodians of a special field of knowledge acquired by long, assiduous study, and they are respected and accorded privileges because of that fact. Second, it is a loose grouping of individuals rather than a pyramidal organization. The true profession is a voluntary binding together of independent members, deriving none of their sustenance from the association, utterly uncontrolled in their thoughts and actions as long as they remain within the law and within the code of the association itself. Third, every profession has, to some degree a symbolism and ritual of its own. Fourth, there is often, especially in the older professions, a means of maintaining standards and for disciplining those who violate a code, usually backed up by the civil law. Something of the sort is essential, for every profession is surrounded by Charlatans and human nature being what it is, special privileges are bound to be abused. [1957, p. 51]

INTRINSIC AND EXTRINSIC THREATS TO PROFESSIONAL STATURE

Perhaps our greatest challenges to acquiring and maintaining our professionalism today relate to internal and external factors impacting our profession and the persons we serve. Intrinsically, we must recognize ourselves as professionals and accept the rights and responsibilities of being a professional. As a profession, the main purpose of audiology is the provision of quality hearing and balance care to benefit society and improve the conditions under which we live as individuals and groups of individuals. We must base our work on knowledge gained through the process of scientific inquiry and, perhaps, coupled with sound tradition and experience. As a profession, we must assure that we stay within the bounds of our own scope of training and competence. We must make our services available to all persons. We must adhere to a reasonable and progressive code of ethics and recognize the person best qualified to judge our work is another audiologist. Audiology must adhere to a standard of practice and excellence that is based upon knowledge, character, and achievement. As a profession, audiology must work in the best interests of persons with hearing and balance disorders and the professions with which it cooperates. Audiology must offer its membership the right to provide services to whom they please, at the time and price they choose, while they are consistent with the *Code of Ethics of the American Academy of Audiology* (see pp. xv–xxi of this book), laws of the land, and public interest. We must recognize that audiologists have the knowledge and skills to provide quality hearing and balance care services and make decisions independent of the pressure exerted by those outside the profession (Freeman, 1997).

Loh (2000) notes that professionalism is threatened externally by technological advancements that may reduce the role of health-care practitioners in the diagnosis and management of patients, creating more of a technician role for practitioners. The specialization of practitioners may lead to the identification of patients by diagnosis, potentially resulting in impersonal care. Another external threat is the consolidation and corporatization of health care with more emphasis on corporate profits than on patient care. Professionals are susceptible to the potential for, or a patient perception of, practitioner greed, which can lead to a lack of patient trust.

BUILDING AND MAINTAINING PROFESSIONALISM

Practitioners are measured by every professional and nonprofessional contact. Whether self-employed or an employee, professional and personal habits reflect on our profession. The public, employers, and referral sources measure practitioners by their appearance, clinical facilities, practice and interpersonal skills, and professional status in the community. As a profession, we can control and direct the extrinsic view of audiology by displaying a thorough knowledge and application of our literature, along with the character to merit the confidence of the public and other professionals.

It is critical that audiologists avoid negative patient perceptions and remain focused on building patient trust in our knowledge and skills. Professional autonomy lies in the responsibility placed on us by our education and stature within a community. Audiologists must assume responsibility and recognize the value of our contributions to the health and welfare of our patients. We must communicate on a personal and professional level with other health-care providers and become involved in community and professional activities while adhering to our *Code of Ethics*.

REFERENCES

Bean WB. (1968) *Sir William Osler: Aphorisms from His Bedside Teachings and Writings*. Springfield, IL: Charles C. Thomas.

Bush V. (1957) Professional collaboration. *Science* 125(3237):49–54.

Freeman BA. (1997) The meaning of professionalism. *Audiol Today* 9(1):7–8.

Loh K. (2000) Professionalism, where are you? *Ear Nose Throat J* 79(4):242–246.

business are commercial enterprises that involve providing goods + svcs —involvg fin, comm. & industrial aspects. Has NO COE; no morals; no emotions.

Chapter 3

Approaches to Analyzing Ethical Dilemmas
Carol Fleisher, Certificate in Clinical Bioethics

Many of the things we do in life—our personal daily choices and actions, even our thoughts—are determined by moral evaluations. We are moral beings who recognize right and wrong and who choose or refuse certain actions. In professional life, moral and ethical considerations are of great importance. As health-care professionals, we have information, decision-making power, and authority status that patients do not. In addition, those seeking care are commonly sick, distressed, fearful, or worried. This creates a significant imbalance between provider and patient, an imbalance in which vulnerable patients need special ethical protection. This requires that health-care professionals assume certain ethical responsibilities.

The health-care industry is a complex set of moral cross-currents involving many participants, many interests, and many conflicting motivations and incentives. Health-care professionals face issues of truth telling, integrity, advocacy, fraud, confidentiality, self-interest, honesty, fairness, informed consent, loyalty, whistle-blowing, prestige, commercialization, and so on. For these reasons, health-care professionals need a well-developed awareness of ethical issues and an effective process for making good decisions. This chapter will describe the key elements of a decision-making framework for recognizing and analyzing professional ethical issues. The basic moral concepts that can be used in resolving ethical dilemmas will be discussed.

MORALS, VALUES, AND ETHICS

Morality refers to beliefs about right and wrong human conduct that transcend time and are so widely shared they fashion a communal consensus (Smedes, 1991). These binding common beliefs form moral obligations or duties. Moral rules are learned alongside social rules and laws beginning in early childhood, and they establish the conduct one "ought" to take. The concept of "ought" is the essence of morality. "Ought" refers to what one is obliged to do by moral duty, such as to impart benefit or at least do no harm, to be honest, and so forth. *vs.*

In contrast to morals, values are personally held and culturally based. Values are subjective. The value or worth one individual places on some thing or some action may be more or less than that of another individual.

Professional codes of ethics are the rules and principles that govern the behavior of the members of a profession. They are based on the morals and values of the professional members and are statements of the principles that patients and other professionals expect us to uphold.

ETHICAL CONFLICTS AND DILEMMAS

An "ethical dilemma" is a situation in which two equally weighted moral obligations are in conflict; one obligation has to be set aside. Some have said that true ethical dilemmas are very rare. Most of the time we know what is morally right, what action ought to trump all other actions. Resolving a true ethical dilemma requires a difficult choice—one of the two moral obligations cannot be honored. Ethical dilemmas can arise between individuals (e.g., a patient and a professional) or within an individual.

Personal conflicts are more common than true ethical dilemmas. When competing values are in conflict, the situation begs for the "right" answer. These situations create an internal conflict or personal dilemma, rather than a true ethical dilemma. The tension between self-interest and altruism is a common source of personal dilemmas. Self-interest, for material possessions, pleasure, or status, can be a compelling force. Today's health-care arena has no shortage of self-interest enticements. They can come from manufacturers or be in the form of political advantage, prestige, or sexual favors. Conflicts between self-interests (including fraud and other incentives) may create temptation, especially when placing self-interest over ethical obligations does not violate any legal obligations and falls within the realm of culturally acceptable behaviors. Edmond Pellegrino addressed the subject of self-interest when he wrote, "we are all too good at rationalizing what we want to do so personal gain can be converted from vice to virtue" (1999, p. 46). In our present time, self-gain is considered acceptable, and frequently there is peer pressure to pursue self-gain. Medical professionals must adhere to higher standards or risk the loss of trust of patients and other medical professionals.

Ethical and personal dilemmas do not routinely present themselves in a straightforward manner. Often a dilemma is enveloped within a multitude of contextual circumstances that cloud the opposing moral or ethical obligations. Approaching a dilemma systematically and methodically provides a starting point for reducing conflict and facilitating resolution. This process involves (1) identifying the dilemma, (2) collecting and analyzing relevant information, (3) framing the issues, (4) deliberating, and (5) evaluating and reflecting.

IDENTIFYING THE DILEMMA

When dilemmas occur, one has to first identify the nature of the conflict. Professional-patient relationships can give rise to ethical dilemmas that revolve around privacy, truth telling, confidentiality, advocacy, or informed consent. Informed consent dilemmas may arise while caring for minors or for individuals whose cognition is compromised as a result of age, trauma, or disease. An individual, such as an elderly adult, may be *legally* competent to give informed consent to the purchase of a hearing aid, for example, but may lack the decision-making capacity to do so. It may not be ethical for an audiologist to assume that the patient can act in his or her own best interest. The first step in resolving a dilemma is to identify the dilemma and ethical or moral obligations. Moral dilemmas are not easily recognized and not easily resolved.

COLLECTING AND ANALYZING RELEVANT INFORMATION

Facts, Fallacies, and Notions

It can be helpful to list the facts of the case and determine whether some are actually fallacies or notions. When the facts are known and understood, it may become clear that values or moral obligations are not in conflict, as originally assumed.

Do all parties agree on the language and terms? One party may define an action in a manner that makes it inconsistent with his or her own moral code, while the other party equates the definition with a morally appropriate action (Beauchamp and Walters, 1999). By way of illustration, the moral controversy in the dilemma surrounding the removal of life-sustaining treatment hinges on whether removal means "allowing natural death" or "killing." For audiologists, terms such as "confidentiality," "appropriate patient care," "professional competence," "conflict of interest," "supervision," "exploitation," "research," and "dishonesty" may need to be clearly defined before a decision can be made.

Philosopher David Hume noted that nonmoral elements such as emotions may be intense (Hume, [1751]1987). Consider, for example, that love and hate have launched ships and initiated wars. Emotions and notions regarding motives or personal agendas complicate situations between disputing parties. These elements are human responses generated by concerns about the nature of the situation and must be acknowledged if resolution of the situation is to occur. Humans respond to what they perceive. If one party perceives an ulterior motive by the other, then a trusting relationship is absent, and the process cannot proceed to meaningful deliberation. Emotional responses can give rise to fallacies and notions that can block resolution of dilemmas.

Culturally appropriate communication that recognizes ethnic and religious influences and traditions is essential when dealing with emotions and notions. Calm and sincere communication needs to be sensitive to the situation, the surroundings, and the individuals involved. Meaningful interaction demonstrates caring and builds a shared understanding between conflicting parties. Caring has a cognitive dimension; it provides insight into circumstances, needs, and feelings of the parties involved (Beauchamp and Childress, 1994).

Determining Applicable Guidelines, Ethical Principles, and Legal Constraints

After identifying the particular circumstances of the dilemma that need to be resolved, the next step is to place the circumstances in their proper perspective. The audiologist should review position statements, guidelines, and the American Academy of Audiology's *Code of Ethics* (see pp. xv–xxi of this book) to identify the shared beliefs and values of the profession. Position statements on standard of care may also be relevant, if the issue involves a question of quality of patient care. Because of the fiduciary relationship between professional and patient, a relationship in which power is entrusted to the professional, a higher level of conduct is demanded. The specific knowledge and skills of the audiologist set him or her apart from others and underpin the trusting relationship with patients. The audiologist should ensure that a professional standard of care is consistently delivered. Although every situation cannot be addressed by reviewing relevant documents, these statements serve to protect and preserve the integrity of the profession and the professional and may provide insight and guidance.

Negative consequences can be imposed for activities outside legal boundaries. It is important to understand current laws governing the practice of audiology, including the educational requirements, scope of practice, fraud, abuse, and other legislated or regulated areas. Since laws reflect normative societal values, they are dynamic and change with cases; thus, case law becomes important. Likewise, professionals have a responsibility to work through appropriate channels to change laws and regulations whenever the need arises; they are not free to disregard the laws with which they do not agree.

Relevant institutional policies should also be consulted. Health-care organizations generally have policies on conflict of interest and oftentimes have ethical boards that can assist in decision making.

Sometimes the nature of the dilemma is fully identified in this manner and a course of action is suggested. Other times the dilemma's resolution is not found in societal codes and advisory statements. In these cases, more fact-finding is required.

Players and Stakeholders

Successfully resolving a dilemma may also entail a clear understanding of just who the involved parties and stakeholders are. Primary players are directly involved in the dilemma and in deciding which action one should take. Stakeholders ultimately share in the benefits or burdens resulting from the action taken. Generally, a fiscal or fiduciary relationship exists between players and stakeholders. Primary players have a vested interest in the dilemma and actively participate in the deliberation process. Secondary players have the power to influence the primary players even after the dilemma has culminated into an action. While secondary players hold no personal stake in the situation, attention to their role promotes a more stable and lasting environment overall. Listing the players and stakeholders, and ensuring that the views of each are understood, can help clarify the situation.

Consideration of the Time Frame

Deliberating the choice of action requires time. Considering the effects of delaying decisions, and balancing them with the consequences of making rushed decisions, are also appropriate steps in the information collection process.

Helpful Questions

Monsignor Fahey (1995), Executive Director of Fordham University's Third Age Center, provided the following questions, which may prove useful in collecting and analyzing information.
- What are the influences at work, and how do they appropriately or inappropriately enter into the decision-making process and affect its outcome?
- Why is a decision necessary?
- What is at stake and for whom? What is the decision's significance?
- Will the decision be temporary or permanent?
- What is the cost, financial or otherwise, of the proposed solutions?
- How profoundly will the decision affect the stakeholders' well-being— physical, psychological, and spiritual?
- Who should be involved in the deliberation? With whom should the final decision-making authority reside?

FRAMING THE ISSUE

The specifics of the situation should be systematically peeled back to the foundation of the dilemma, allowing the points of controversy to be identified and to more fully frame the dilemma. When the issues and their contextual matters have been identified, and the emotions and notions have been addressed, one can begin to frame the dilemma. Framing is the process of constructing a clear picture of the dilemma from an analysis of its constituent parts. With the contextual matters peeled away, the conflicting moral and ethical obligations should be recognized. In the case of true ethical dilemmas, the conflicting "oughts" would then be clearly defined. One should then be able to identify the rationale in support of each of the competing obligations

DELIBERATION

"Deliberation" is a process of reasoning in order to formulate a justifiable choice of action. Some of the procedures that can be applied in deliberation are discussed below. There is no absolute right or wrong theory to use when deciding on a course of action, just as there is no absolute right or wrong choice among equally balanced moral obligations. The use of more than one of the approaches described below takes the level of discourse above that of mediation or a simple consensus of personal opinions. Different approaches may point to distinctly different resolutions.

Each course of action will result in a consequence, outcome, and effect. As with a stone cast into a lake, the immediate splash is inevitably accompanied by ripples. Therefore, the consequences of each course of action must be considered for both immediate *and* future effect on the involved players as well as the stakeholders. Focusing on the consequences leads one to ask such questions as: What physical, spiritual, material, and psychosocial benefits will result? Who will reap the benefits? What burdens will be imposed? Will the burdens be physical or financial? Will there be a negative impact on relationships, a compromise to the integrity of the profession or, more broadly, will there be a negative impact on society as a whole? What risks are involved? What weight does each of these carry? Consequences are unavoidable and important; thus, it is prudent to seek positive consequences. As King Midas discovered, one must be mindful of unintended consequences. For example, there are unintended consequences when an audiologist persuasively recommends amplification to an elderly patient who is too proud to acknowledge that there is insufficient money to purchase groceries, medication, and amplification.

Utilitarian Approach to Dilemmas

A utilitarian approach renders a decision based on providing the "greatest good to the greatest number of people." This focus on the consequences of the decision makes utilitarianism a pragmatic approach. After a comparative evaluation of the consequences for each of the possible alternatives, the "right" decision is the alternative that provides the greatest good and the least burden without regard to the means utilized to achieve the results. Clearly, a good outcome has natural appeal. But utilitarianism is not without limitations. Against what measurement is "the greatest good" determined? To whom are the burdens assigned? Decision makers must guard against being seduced by the means to achieve a good outcome. Care must be taken not to allow the end to justify the means.

Rights-/Duty-Based or Legalist Ethics

Legalist ethics draws completely and specifically on the constitution. It holds that moral norms reflect the consensus of the majority and are codified in legislation and the constitution (Joint Commission on Accreditation of Healthcare Organizations, 1998). Individual rights and entitlements are priorities, based on the concept of liberty. Professionals have a legal duty to impart benefit or fulfill the contractual responsibilities as required by local, state, and federal laws. Failure of a professional to fulfill the duties ascribed by law is considered a breach and can be the basis for a malpractice suit. This ethic supports informed consent or informed refusal and other such actions rooted in individual liberty. Both respect for the law and consideration of any legal precedent is important, but this ethic falls short in its scope of ethical inquiry. Decisions are often rendered defensively, out of fear for the potential negative legal consequences.

Casuistry

Casuistry, or case-based reasoning, relies on practical wisdom and well-developed perception to guide morality (Kuczewski, 1997). Casuistry builds on arguments for or against ethical principles utilized in previous or similar cases. This form of ethical inquiry does not focus on universal principles or duties; instead, it looks for relevant precedents in other cases and determines how each applies to the specific case at hand in much the same way the judicial system develops case law. Casuistry provides some measure of assurance regarding consistency, but it is susceptible to the changes in societal norms that are reflected in paradigm cases.

Deontological Approach

Duty-based, or, more appropriately, deontological, ethical decision making is based on unchanging moral precepts regardless of the consequences. As expressed by Aristotle, "ethos," the Greek word from which "ethics" is derived, is "moral character" reflected in a "deliberate choice of action developed into a habit of mind" (1987). Moral precepts such as right, and good, and truth obligate us to intentionally choose virtues over vices and develop these into habits and character traits, leading one to make decisions and take action based on these unchanging duties. By any standard, a virtuous person does what is right and good consistently—even when no one is watching.

Virtue ethics establishes a logical progression of this theory. Virtues that are developed into traits in one's character are founded in timeless moral precepts. As such, honesty, truthfulness, fairness, trustworthiness, loyalty, faithfulness, devotion, dependability, and other virtues become moral duties the virtuous individual owes others and self. Moral duties, then, are an implicit part of veracity, humility, and fidelity. Ethical conduct is the active expressive fulfillment of these duties.

Consideration of Beneficence, Nonmaleficence, Justice, and Patient Autonomy

The principles of autonomy, beneficence, nonmaleficence, and justice are frequently applied in the arena of health care. "Autonomy" recognizes that individuals have volition, will, and, except in certain circumstances, are capable of self-direction. Acknowledging that individuals have an inherent right to make choices, hold views, and act based on their own belief systems and values demonstrates respect for the dignity and worth of every individual. "Beneficence" is the ethical obligation to act for the benefit of others (Beauchamp and Childress, 1994). "Beneficence" can extend further to include other concepts such as charity and kindness. "Nonmaleficence" is refraining from inflicting intentional harm on others and is frequently expressed as "do no harm." "Justice," although not easily defined, encompasses the idea of fairness within a set of conditions. Autonomy, beneficence, nonmaleficence, and justice are ethical obligations. These principles serve as the cornerstone for most health-care professionals' guidelines for conduct and formal codes of ethics, and differ from mere legal obligations. Deliberation should entail efforts to apply different approaches in reaching a solution to the dilemma. The final course of action must be morally and ethically justifiable.

EVALUATING AND REFLECTING

Evaluation is the learning process that allows us to grow, improve, and subsequently to share that which was learned. It is worthwhile to evaluate the resolution, or the reason for the dilemma not being adequately resolved. Resolution between parties is more likely if agreement on a common set of ethical guidelines can be utilized. However, in a society with multiple values, beliefs, and rules, consensus about what is right or wrong is frequently lacking. Values are inherently subjective and specific to an individual even though they are founded in moral precepts. Resolution may not occur when there is a significant value disparity between parties.

Reflection is too often omitted from the process, yet reflecting on these weighty issues allows one to sort through, consider, and contemplate them in preparation for future dilemmas.

SAMPLE CASE

As an example, the following case will be analyzed to illustrate the steps that one may take in analyzing and resolving an ethical dilemma: An audiologist in a busy medical practice is serving as preceptor for a fourth-year Au.D. student. It is Friday at 4:00 p.m. The other licensed audiologist has left early, having no scheduled patients, and the ENT physicians are out of the office. The last case of the day—a four-year-old child—arrives. What had not been noted in the schedule is that this new patient is developmentally delayed and hyperactive. The child's mother seems particularly stressed and anxious. The reception staff has made comments to each other within the audiologist's earshot indicating that they hope that they will be able to leave by 5:00 p.m., particularly since it is Friday.

Testing begins with both the preceptor and student participating in play audiometry. The student is with the child in the sound booth, assisting the child in the play audiometry task and is doing well in managing the child's behavior. The receptionist comes in asking to see the audiologist immediately. The Chief Executive Officer (CEO) of the adjacent hospital is in the waiting room. In a hasty consultation with the walk-in patient, the audiologist learns that the CEO had a minor head trauma two days earlier and since has experienced dizziness when turning his head. He has just been seen by the neurologist in the medical office building, who recognized the symptoms of benign paroxysmal positional vertigo (BPPV) but lacked the expertise in treatment and therefore referred him to the audiologist. As the audiologist asks the CEO to please wait another 15–30 minutes while the audiologist and doctoral student finish testing the child, the CEO explains that he has a flight to catch at 6:30, and has, at most, 30 minutes before he must leave the office. He will be away for a week and is significantly disabled by his symptoms.

Identifying the Ethical Dilemmas

This scenario revolves around resource utilization, as well as commitments to patients, students, and staff. Often the term "scarce resources" is thought of on a grand scale such as insufficient organs to meet transplant needs, or insufficient money to cover the ever-increasing number of services reimbursed by Medicare or Medicaid. Resources, particularly scarce resources, must be distributed in a just manner, consistent with the shared standards of the profession. In this scenario the audiologist is confronted with a dilemma of how to distribute services in a just manner given the time constraints.

The particulars in this case can be peeled back to reveal the issues, starting with staff issues, which constitute a small, but separate, conflict. Is the support staff required to work late if the professional staff must? Relevant information would include staff contracts and perhaps investigation into the consequences of the staff working late. It may be appropriate to allow the most involved stakeholders—the staff themselves—to become the players who make the decision. A utilitarian approach to this small conflict would favor the resolution that inconveniences the fewest. Those favoring a legalist approach or casuistry would be primarily concerned with acting in a way that is consistent with the job description of the staff. The beneficent audiologist would assure the support staff they can leave on time, and the audiologist would assume any extra burden personally.

While the fundamental concern in the central dilemma is equitable utilization of the audiologic resources, there may be concerns about self-gain that might occur by ingratiating oneself to the CEO of the hospital. The unscheduled patient is referred to by job title rather than name. Founded in a long-standing social contract applicable to all health-care disciplines is the recognition that every individual is of equal worth. Therefore, care is rendered based on medical criteria regardless of an individual's station in life, age, race, religion, or any other factor. Referring to patients by their name reduces even the appearance of discrimination or any other form of impropriety. Absent his name, we will refer to him as "Mr. Smith" to reflect the importance of considering the patient's need for service, rather than his status and its potential influence on the audiologist.

The audiologist and the student both freely accepted the profession's commitment to service, including putting patients' needs above their own. Professionalism dictates that both should continue to provide all their services past 5:00 p.m., if required, so this issue has been peeled away.

Collecting and Analyzing Information

Mr. Smith and the pediatric patient and his mother are stakeholders. At this point, something is known about what follows next in the day for Mr. Smith (he has a plane to board) but not for other involved parties. Insufficient information can taint perceptions and lead to assumptions that may not be valid. For example, suppose the mother is a brittle diabetic and needs to return home by 5:30 p.m. for an insulin injection; or suppose the mother is a member of the city council or a school board and has a 6:00 p.m. meeting to attend; or suppose the child has a scheduled activity intended to enhance development. The mother and/or the child may have obligations that are as meaningful within the context of their own lives or the lives of others as boarding a plane is to Mr. Smith. Mr. Smith may be taking a discretionary trip that could be readily postponed. Further fact-finding is required.

Consideration of standards and codes would be required. Is there sufficient time to treat Mr. Smith successfully? Will the standard of care be reduced in order to treat the patient within the available time? Has the patient been informed of the risks, including the risks that the time available will be exceeded or the condition worsened if, for example, the otolithic debris were to migrate to the horizontal canal?

The audiologist accepted the role of preceptor and has an obligation to fulfill that duty regardless of the capabilities of the student or the complexity of any case. What are the student's needs for professional experience? Is the student able to care for either case independently without compromising quality of care? The *Code of Ethics* requires appropriate supervision. State law or insurance reimbursement rules may prohibit independent student service provision. Given the complexity of each case, it would appear unlikely that the appropriate resolution to the solution would be to have the student assume the primary responsibility for either patient. If, however, the student is able to care for one or both patients, it is then relevant to ask whether the student would benefit most from the experience in working with one or both patients. The preceptor is responsible not only for teaching the technical aspects of the field of audiology, but he or she is also responsible for teaching the student how to act professionally.

Framing the Issue

The four-year-old developmentally delayed and hyperactive child had a scheduled appointment and testing is underway. Thus, the professional-patient relationship has been established. The mother is no doubt anxious to obtain information about her child. Both mother and child had to prepare for the visit and arrived for their appointment in a responsible manner. Absent other overriding circumstances, this would appear to be the central issue in the resolution. The dilemma demands that this primary obligation to provide service to this patient be honored. Mr. Smith, anxious to leave for his flight and anxious over his own condition, has given the audiologist "at most" 30 minutes. This may be an insufficient period of time to achieve the desired outcome. Utilitarianism would favor providing service to both patients if that course of action is feasible; however, there are concerns about quality of care and appropriate student supervision.

Deliberation

There are many approaches to resolving the dilemma, some more satisfactory than others. A legalist approach to the dilemma would hold that Mr. Smith is not yet accepted as a patient and thus is not entitled to the same level of care as is the child. However, refusing to provide services is in conflict with the tenet of beneficence that underlies the health-care professions.

The utilitarian approach focuses on the course of action that provides the greatest good. If it is possible for the mother to assist with play audiometry with the student conducting the testing, then the audiologist will be free to treat Mr. Smith. Alternatively, if the student is experienced in BPPV evaluation and treatment, the student could assume care of Mr. Smith. It is assumed that the ethic of truth telling will prompt the audiologist to be forthright with the patients—either in telling the mother that the student will complete the testing independently, or by telling Mr. Smith that he will be treated with indirect supervision by the student. Having the student work with only indirect supervision allows the team to provide more patient care but may be untenable for a variety of reasons. This potential solution minimizes the importance of the training needs of the student. The audiologist cannot completely fulfill his or her duty as preceptor if the student acts independently. Likewise, the student could learn from participating in the care of each of these cases.

Additionally, it is unclear whether the student will be able to provide appropriately complex care autonomously. Rights-/duty-based considerations and legal standards should be considered. The child's appointment, a contract for service, was made with the audiologist as a professional. The potential for legal ramifications should also be noted. If testing/treatment is not performed appropriately, malpractice may occur. Billing for services rendered by the student without direct supervision may not be legal.

Deontological or duty-based ethics, coupled with the virtues of truthfulness and fairness, suggest that open and honest communication with the involved parties is appropriate. There are two potential ways of resolving the dilemma via mediated communication. Mr. Smith could be encouraged to reschedule his flight for a later time, and in so doing, adequate time would be available to provide the services he needs. He would then be seen for evaluations and potential treatment by the audiologist after the child's evaluation is complete. Without treatment, Mr. Smith will likely remain disabled by his symptoms, and this information should be disclosed to him. The risks and benefits of treatment, as well the risks and benefits of no treatment, should be disclosed in every case. Alternatively, the mother, on behalf of the child, may be willing to interrupt testing until Mr. Smith receives complete care. All parties should be advised that the process may take longer than 30 minutes. Again, risks, benefits, and burdens imposed should be disclosed to all parties prior to any decisions. In both these situations, the patients are cared for at different time intervals with both preceptor and student involved in each case. However, one or the other patient is by necessity inconvenienced.

Evaluating and Reflecting

Reflecting on such cases allows one to see with greater clarity the issues, duties, potential risks and benefits, and other available options in a different light. In the hectic day-to-day activities associated with professional life, it is wise to pause, reflect, and approach duties in a considered and deliberated manner. This is particularly true in this case, where by necessity, a decision must be reached in mere minutes.

Dilemmas, by their very nature, relegate us to choosing only one path to walk down when many are available. As illustrated in this case, there is no solution that does not have an adverse impact on one or more of the parties. Here, the student and preceptor would both gain from post hoc discussion of the various means of resolving the dilemma, their feelings about the outcome, and whether, in retrospect, a different decision might have been preferable. The student stands to improve his or her audiologic skills through mentored experience with either or both patients but will learn a more important professional lesson by seeing how this patient-care dilemma is resolved.

SUMMARY

The study of ethics provides insight into the ways in which ethical dilemmas can be solved. Careful analysis of the nature of the dilemma at hand and consideration of a variety of solutions increases the likelihood of a good outcome. Audiologists personally stand to gain from deliberately approaching dilemmas—careful resolution of conflicts helps to ensure a good night's sleep. As discussed by Freeman in this volume (see Chapter 2), failure to act in an ethical manner erodes professional stature. The profession benefits when professionals resolve the dilemmas in keeping with the traditions of the health-care professions; it demonstrates the accountability and high ethical standards of the profession.

REFERENCES

Aristotle. (1987) *The Nicomachean Ethics*. Trans. Welldon JEC. New York: Promethius Books.

Beauchamp TL, Childress J. (1994) *Principles of Biomedical Ethics*. 4th ed. New York: Oxford University Press.

Beauchamp TL, Walters L. (1999) *Contemporary Issues in Bioethics*. 5th ed. Belmont, CA: Wadsworth Publishing Company.

Fahey C. (1995) American Health Care Association Conference Presentation.

Hume D. ([1751]1987) A treatise of human nature: a dialog. In: *An Enquiry Concerning the Principles of Morals*. Vol. 35 of *Great Books of the Western World*. Chicago: Encyclopedia Britannica, 465–466.

Joint Commission on Accreditation of Healthcare Organizations. (1998) *Ethical Issues and Patient Rights: Across the Continuum of Care*. Oakbrook Terrace, IL: Joint Commission on Accreditation of Healthcare Organizations.

Kuczewski M. (1997) *Fragmentation and Consensus: Communitarian and Casuist Bioethics*. Washington, DC: Georgetown University Press.

Pellegrino E. (1999) The virtuous physician and the ethics of medicine. In: Beauchamp TL, Walters L, eds. *Contemporary Issues in Bioethics*. 5th ed. Belmont, CA: Wadsworth Publishing Company, 46–51.

Smedes L. (1991) *Choices: Making Right Decisions in a Complex World*. San Francisco: Harper-Collins.

Chapter 4

Relationships with Hearing Instrument Manufacturers

David Hawkins, Ph.D.
Marilyn Larkin, Au.D.
Thomas J. Tedeschi, Au.D.

The history of the relationship between audiologists and hearing instrument manufacturers is interesting and varied. When audiology began as a profession in the 1940s, all hearing aids were dispensed by a hearing aid sales force, which did not include audiologists. Audiologists were primarily located in universities, hospitals, and community speech and hearing centers and were not directly involved in the dispensing of any type of amplification device. Those dispensing hearing aids, at the time called "hearing aid dealers," were viewed by the hearing instrument manufacturers as a sales force, part of a distribution system similar to any other commercial product.

The role of audiologists in the hearing aid distribution system was limited, as the *Code of Ethics* of the American Speech and Hearing Association (ASHA) prohibited audiologists from being engaged in the sale of a device. As a result, the audiologist's involvement originally consisted of evaluating stock behind-the-ear hearing aids on patients in a clinical setting. These hearing aids were loaned to the audiologist by the manufacturers and were considered "consignment aids." The audiologist typically tested speech discrimination (word recognition) in a sound booth with several different models in order to arrive at a specific model recommendation. The patient was then referred to a local hearing aid dealer to purchase the aid(s) that provided the best performance in the clinical test environment. In some cases, the patient returned to the audiologist to verify that appropriate aided performance was being obtained, but the majority of follow-up was performed by the hearing aid dealer. As a result, the audiologist never purchased hearing aids from the manufacturers, and there were no financial relationships between audiologists and manufacturers. All financial dealings were between the manufacturers and the hearing aid dealer sales force. Additionally, hearing aid dealers sold products to patients who did not utilize the services of an audiologist, placing the dealers directly in the sales arena. As with any sales force of a product, a variety of incentives were offered to exact a measure of brand loyalty and to increase purchases. Hearing aids were not viewed as a health-care device but a commercial product to be sold on the market, and hence, the incentives were offered to encourage sales.

In the late 1970s, ASHA removed the prohibition against audiologists dispensing a product for profit. The *Code of Ethics* of ASHA was changed to reflect the practice of hearing aid dispensing by audiologists. Suddenly, the hearing instrument manufacturers had two groups in the distribution system: hearing aid dealers and audiologists. The manufacturers did not view the two groups as different in terms of financial relationships. The same sales incentives that had been offered to hearing aid dealers were now offered to the new dispensing audiologist. Cruises, trips, cash rebates, and other incentives were sometimes offered and accepted by both groups. Very few audiologists realized at the time that acceptance of such incentives violated the conflict of interest statement in ASHA's *Code of Ethics*. Initially, however, very few audiologists were involved in the direct dispensing of hearing aids, and since the sales incentives were not well publicized, there was no obvious concern expressed within the professional organization about the ethical implications of the incentive system.

It is clear that the relationship between the audiologist and the hearing instrument manufacturer is an extremely important one. Today, the majority of audiologists dispense hearing aids directly to their patients and thus maintain a financial relationship with a number of hearing instrument companies. It is important that the audiologists structure these relationships in a way that is practical and profitable to their practice and yet consistent with the ethical guidelines outlined by their professional associations. Recently, the American Academy of Audiology (Academy) and the Academy of Dispensing Audiologists have issued several statements that clarify ethical implications of many aspects of the financial relationships between audiologists and hearing instrument manufacturers. The purpose of this chapter is to provide some context for these statements and give examples of how they are applied to everyday decision making.

EVOLUTION OF THE POSITION OF THE AMERICAN ACADEMY OF AUDIOLOGY ON CONFLICTS OF INTEREST

Audiology was not the only profession to evaluate the ethics of incentives provided to its members. Pharmaceutical manufacturers were able to track physician dispensing and reward those who favored their prescription brands with trips, disproportionate honoraria, and other incentives. The American Medical Association (AMA) created guidelines on "Gifts to Physicians from Industry" in 1992 to curtail these practices in order to avoid potential loss of physician/patient trust, and to ensure that members acted within legal confines (American Medical Association, Council on Ethical and Judicial Affairs, 2004). Communication between pharmaceutical representatives and physicians continues; however, the framework of the relationship was modified by these guidelines. Similarly, the Academy has evaluated the issues surrounding various financial relationships with manufacturers in light of its established *Code of Ethics (COE;* see pp. xv–xxi of this book).

The Academy *COE* has a simple and very straightforward statement regarding professional conflicts of interest. Rule 4c states: "Individuals shall not participate in activities that constitute a conflict of professional interest." While this rule has been in existence since the inception of the Academy in 1988, it had received little attention as to how it should be interpreted in light of relationships with instrument manufacturers. Both David Resnick and, later, Newell Decker (former chairs of the Academy Ethical Practice Board [EPB] during the early years of the association) wrote about this topic in "Issues in Ethics" statements published in *Audiology Today.* Decker offered the following recommendations:

> The Ethical Practices Board should take a strong stand against conflict of interest, including a revision of the present, rather weak, Conflict of Interest statement. Second, the EPB, in concert with the AAA Board of Directors, should appoint a task force made up of AAA members as well as representatives from industry to study the interface between the professional and the manufacturer and the potential conflicts that arise from that interface. In my view the outcome of that task force ought to be a recommendation and an agreement to stop the ever escalating industry convention room parties, the excessive expenditures on opening night parties, and to put an end to incentive plans of all kinds.... Third, each audiologist is honor bound to hold strictly to the rules surrounding the Code of Ethics of either or both ASHA and AAA. To do anything less is a gross disregard for the very essence of our profession.... In closing, let me quote from the Academy's 1997 position statement on Conflict of Interest: "Society recognizes audiologists as professionals. This means that audiologists accept a fiduciary and ethical responsibility to scrutinize the purpose, appearance, and ramifications of all offers of gifts and other types of support to ensure that their acceptance does not create, or appear to create, a potential conflict of professional interest. By assuming these fiduciary and ethical responsibilities, audiologists protect their independent judgment, maintain their professional dignity, and preserve public confidence in the profession of audiology." [1999, p. 29]

Just as concern was being expressed in the audiology community, the AMA became aware that some physicians and industry representatives were not adhering to the published guidelines on gift giving. In response, the AMA and pharmaceutical companies jointly agreed in 2000 to initiate an educational effort to raise awareness of the guidelines among physicians (American Medical Association, 2004). In the audiology arena, David Fabry, then president of the Academy, appointed a Presidential Task Force in 2001 to study conflicts of interest with product manufacturers. Brian Walden, of Walter Reed Army Medical Center, chaired the task force, which produced a document making a number of recommendations to the Academy Board of Directors regarding this issue. The recommendations of the task force were passed to the subsequent president of the Academy, Angela Loavenbruck, who became actively involved in educating the membership of the need for new guidelines for conflicts of interest. In addition, she helped to forge an alliance with the Academy of Dispensing Audiologists (ADA). Loavenbruck made the issue a central theme of her presidency and frequently presented on the topic of how the privileges of professional autonomy require avoidance of even the appearance of a conflict of interest. In 2003, a document was approved by the board of directors of both associations and was published in *Audiology Today*. This document, *Ethical Practice Guidelines on Financial Incentives from Hearing Instrument Manufacturers*, hereafter called the *Ethical Practice Guidelines*, is reprinted in full in Appendix 1.

The key underlying tenet in the *Ethical Practice Guidelines* is that, in order to avoid the appearance of a conflict of interest, the audiologist should practice in a manner such that the patient's welfare always comes first. If this tenet is followed, the patient will have the utmost confidence in the objectivity of all clinical decisions. There should be nothing in the way that the audiologist deals with products or manufacturers of products that could lead the patient to believe that his or her best interests are not paramount in the audiologist's mind.

ETHICAL RESTRICTIONS VERSUS LEGAL RESTRICTIONS

While this chapter is about ethical issues associated with acceptance of gifts and inducements from manufacturers, audiologists should be aware that accepting such gifts may also violate the law. The federal Anti-Kickback Statute (42 U.S.C. § 1320a-7b) provides that any person who "knowingly and willfully solicits or receives any remuneration (including any kickback, bribe, or rebate) directly or indirectly, overtly or covertly, in cash or in kind ... in return for purchasing, leasing, [or] ordering ... any ... item for which payment may be made in whole or in part under a Federal health care program" is "guilty of a felony." Penalties may include heavy fines, imprisonment, and exclusion from participation in federal health-care programs. It should also be noted that many states have their own state anti-kickback laws, which may differ from the federal Anti-Kickback Statute.

Thus, if an audiologist accepts gifts or other remuneration from a hearing aid manufacturer in return for purchases of that manufacturer's hearing aids, and if the hearing aids are payable under a federal health-care program (e.g., Medicaid), there may be an anti-kickback violation. A prosecutor must show that the remuneration was in return for or to induce purchases, but the prosecutor is only required to show that this was one purpose of the remuneration (not necessarily that it was the only purpose). It is important to note that an audiologist cannot avoid violating the law by informing patients of the gifts or inducements received from manufacturers. That is because the law is not intended only to protect patients from conflicts of interest; it is also designed to protect federal health-care programs from overutilization of reimbursable items and services.

The law provides for some "safe harbors." Acceptance of gifts or inducements that fit within a "safe harbor" is protected from liability. One such "safe harbor" is for discounts that meet the following requirements:

- The discount is a reduction in the amount a buyer is charged for an item or service based on an arms-length transaction;
- The discount is not in the form of a payment of cash or cash equivalents, a warranty, an "up-front rebate," or a reduced price to purchase one product or service in exchange for an agreement to purchase a different product or service; and
- The discount is properly disclosed and accurately reflected in any charges billed to a federal health-care program [42 C.F.R. § 1001.952(h)].

EXAMPLES OF HOW THE CONFLICT OF INTEREST GUIDELINES ARE APPLIED

Audiology is a health-care profession, and, as a result, certain retail marketing practices may not be appropriate, acceptable, or legal. As relationships with manufacturers are forged, the interests of the patient must be kept paramount. Audiologists may be presented with a confusing array of marketing incentives from manufacturers, wholesalers, and employers. Various examples of marketing plans are presented and analyzed below.

Volume Discounts

Discounted prices on hearing instruments are offered by manufacturers and buying groups. Manufacturers may offer direct discounts to the audiologist based on the average volume of units ordered over a period of time. Buying groups offer discounts from a number of manufacturers, based on the total purchasing power of the group. An ethical issue could arise if the audiologist commits in advance to purchase a specific number of units in exchange for a discount.

Scenario 1: Audiologist Jones primarily dispenses three brands of hearing instruments, Brand A, Brand B, and Brand C. Jones purchases Brand A directly from the manufacturer, who offers him a 15 percent volume discount in hopes of continuing business with Jones. The manufacturer of Brand B offers him a 25 percent discount in exchange for a commitment to buy at least five units a month. Brand C hearing instruments he purchases through a buying group at a 20 percent savings.

Discount programs do have the potential to benefit the patient. Discounts are disclosed on the manufacturer's invoice and may be passed on to the patient or third-party payor. In this example, the audiologist felt he was serving his patients' best interest by negotiating the best price on their hearing instruments. Purchasing Brand A directly from the manufacturer at a discount presented no ethical issues.

Not OK However, by making a sales commitment to the manufacturer of Brand B, it may appear that the audiologist has not put the patients' interests first, thus breeching the *Ethical Practice Guidelines*. In this scenario, the patient could perceive that a specific brand was recommended only to ensure a prearranged discount. By purchasing Brand C through a buying group, the audiologist was able to receive a volume discount

OK without a commitment to purchase a specific number of hearing aids.

The federal Anti-Kickback Statute allows for discounts, provided the discount is a reduction in the amount a buyer is charged for an item or service based on an "arm's-length transaction." The discount must be properly disclosed and accurately reflected on the invoice. The discount can be in the form of a credit, rebate, or coupon directly redeemable from the seller; it must not include a cash payment. Additionally, a discount may not be accepted in exchange for an agreement to buy a different product or service.

Accepting discounts from buying groups or manufacturers does not constitute a violation of the Academy *COE* provided the audiologist has not entered into an agreement to purchase a specific product or meet a specific sales goal.

Business Development Plans and Reward Banks

Business development plans and reward banks are incentives offered by some manufacturers and buying groups. The dispenser is rewarded with points or dollars for each hearing instrument purchased. The points or dollars are then banked and can be redeemed at a later date for office equipment, business travel, or products.

> Scenario 2: Audiologist Smith signs up for the JoinUS buying group that offers volume discounts and helps with marketing in her private practice. JoinUS issues 100 points for every hearing instrument purchased through their group, regardless of cost of the unit or manufacturer. The points are banked and can be redeemed at the end of the year for seminars, hearing products, advertising or equipment. Smith signs up for the rewards and plans on earning the points necessary to purchase OAE equipment.

This audiologist mistakenly believed that this arrangement presented no conflict of interest because access to the new equipment would serve to benefit her patients. The audiologist also believed that by purchasing the hearing aid as part of the buying group, the ethical issues inherent in taking a reward directly from a manufacturer were avoided. However, in this case, a patient could realistically question whether amplification was truly needed or if a hearing instrument was recommended in order for the audiologist to obtain new equipment. There is a perception of bias in professional judgment anytime an undisclosed rebate or reward is accepted in exchange for purchasing or recommending a product for a patient.

A central problem with reward plans is that the invoice sent by the manufacturer does not reflect the actual cost of the instrument. A portion of the money paid for the unit was held aside and paid back to the dispenser. The audiologist is thus paid for ordering the instrument. It is reasonable to assume the patient's cost of the hearing instrument is based on the acquisition cost of the unit plus professional fees and practice overhead expenses. In the case of business development plans and rewards, the acquisition cost is not accurately represented. When a hearing instrument purchased through a rewards program is billed to a federal program, it represents a possible violation of the federal Anti-Kickback Statute.

If the audiologist, clinic, or employer receives any reward or benefit in exchange for recommending a product or service, a conflict of interest exists. Reward plans of any type, regardless of how the rewards are used, or to whom they are paid, are in violation of the *Ethical Practice Guidelines*. Whether a buying group issued the reward, or whether it is received directly from a manufacturer, has no bearing.

Manufacturers invest significant time and money in rebate and incentive plans. If audiologists were to refuse these plans, the cost to the manufacturer for marketing the product could potentially be reduced. The audiologist would then be in a position to negotiate the best possible price for the hearing aid, void of all rebates and incentive programs.

Loans

Loans from manufacturers to purchase equipment can create the potential for a conflict of interest. Manufacturers may offer to loan money or provide new equipment to the audiologist and accept a payment schedule for the loan based on a preset number of hearing aids monthly.

Scenario 3: Audiologist Adams was setting up a new private practice and contacted New Sound Hearing Aid Company to establish an account. The sales representative offered to provide the office a new real-ear measurement system that would allow for more exacting hearing aid fittings. Adams was told the equipment loan would be interest free and easily repaid, with a $50 credit being applied to the debt reduction for each hearing instrument purchased.

This audiologist felt the real-ear measurement system would surely benefit his patients. He had used New Sound instruments in the past and felt they provided an excellent product for his patients. Since he already planned to use New Sound Hearing Aid Company's products in his practice, it was his belief that this loan would not compromise his professional judgment in the selection process of hearing aids to be used for patients.

Audiologists are free to obtain loans from any source, as long as the repayment is not tied to product purchases. A loan payment made via hearing instrument purchases represents a reward and should be avoided. If the patients who received hearing aids from audiologist Adams were to become aware of the loan arrangement with New Sound, they could easily believe that New Sound instruments were recommended only to pay his debt; thus, there is the appearance of a conflict of interest.

Loan repayments should only include the debt and appropriate interest and should be cash-only transactions; no additional obligations, such as exclusivity or a commitment to purchase other products, should be tied to the loan. In order to avoid even the perception of a conflict of interest, audiologists are encouraged to obtain financing from recognized lending institutions.

Meetings, Meals, and Manufacturers

Manufacturers are an important source of training to help audiologists stay current with new products and technology. Attending seminars and training courses allows the audiologist to share information with colleagues and product representatives. Meals are frequently included and present no ethical dilemma when part of a bona fide educational program.

> Scenario 4: Best Instruments is prepared to release a new product line of dual microphone instruments. In order to fit these instruments properly, audiologists must be trained in the proper techniques for taking impressions, and in the use of the software system to optimize microphone performance. Training is held at regional locations. The audiologists in the Southeastern United States who have active accounts with Best Instruments are invited to attend. Airfare, lodging, and meals are paid by the manufacturer.

It would be preferable for the audiologist to pay his or her own expenses. However, as there is no promise on the part of the audiologist to purchase this new product, nor are only favored, high-volume accounts invited, the audiologist can ethically attend. If the training were not necessary, if social events such as theater tickets were included, if spousal travel were paid for, or if the lodging and/or meals were lavish, then the audiologist would be placed in a conflict of interest position.

> Scenario 5: ACE Hearing Instrument Company is offering a free three-day educational seminar in Maui, Hawaii. The course agenda includes several well-known presenters and will include a chance to network with the experts at a golf outing on the second day.

no extravagant meals

Educational seminars offered by manufacturers in vacation venues with a social agenda should be viewed as an incentive or reward program. In this scenario, it is reasonable to believe the manufacturer is more interested in building a business relationship than sharing knowledge. A trip to Maui is certainly not modest, and it is not a necessary location for this educational experience.

Trips to a hearing instrument manufacturer's facilities can achieve some useful educational objectives, such as observing the hearing aid fabrication process, recognizing the importance of proper earmold impressions, understanding advances in shell fabrication, learning about software updates, and more. These visits may allow the manufacturer to provide instruction that would not be as cost effective if given on a local level. Therefore, travel to a central location for training is not necessarily prohibited. If participation in the trip is dependent on purchase of the manufacturer's product either before or after the training, a conflict of interest exists.

> Scenario 6: The True Sound Hearing Aid Company is introducing a new shell fabrication process and extends an invitation to tour the manufacturing facility and to learn how this process can enhance hearing aid fittings. Airfare, hotel accommodations, and meals will be paid for by the manufacturer with the agreement to purchase 20 hearing aids using the new shell process over the next three months.

The conflict in this scenario arises with the agreement by the audiologist to purchase 20 hearing aids from True Sound. The purchase agreement implies that there is a cost associated with this trip and that the cost is being offset with the purchase of hearing aids. This cost is then passed on to the consumer because of the agreement to purchase the prescribed number of hearing aids. The above example would be within ethical guidelines if there were not an agreement made to purchase the 20 hearing aids. Educational trips and attendance at training seminars sponsored by manufacturers can be accepted as long as the expenses are modest; however, it is important that the trip is not a reward for having purchased from that company in the past and does not require purchases in the future.

Cruises or Vacation Packages

Some hearing instrument manufacturers may offer to reward the audiologist for sales of hearing aids by providing a cruise or other type of vacation reward as a "thank you" for business. Manufacturers will announce a particular sales incentive such as a cruise or vacation package to a particular destination, and the qualification requirement is to sell a designated number of hearing aids or accumulate a number of points within a specified qualification period.

Scenario 7: The Acme Hearing Aid Company announces the introduction of the newest addition to their product line. As this new product is announced, Acme also announces that they are going to offer a Mediterranean cruise to all audiologists who attain 100 points over the next 12 months from the sales of Acme products. Their newest hearing aid is worth 2 points, and all others are worth 1 point. The audiologist already believes that the Acme Hearing Aid Company has the best hearing aids available, and their newest product simply is the very best. He is already engaged in business with Acme, and attainment of the 100 points will be very easy over the next 12 months, because he is already ordering hearing aids that would put his total in excess of the 100 points.

The audiologist thinks that there would not be a conflict of interest because (1) the patient is being provided with what the audiologist thinks are the best hearing aids available; (2) hearing aids for individuals are not being recommended just to make the "points" because their typical dispensing volume meets the required points; and (3) this is viewed just as an additional reward or "thank you" from the manufacturer, separate from the cost of the hearing aids to the patients.

The basic framework for judging this scenario is found in Guideline 3 of the *Ethical Practice Guidelines*: "Travel expenses, registration fees, or compensation for time to attend meetings, conferences or seminars should not be accepted directly or indirectly from a manufacturer. Trips sponsored by a manufacturer that are solely educational may be accepted, provided the cost of the trip is modest and acceptance of the trip does not reward the audiologist for past sales or commit the audiologist to future purchases" (Appendix 1, p. 118 of this book).

There are a number of issues in the above reward scenario. First, there are costs associated with the trip, which are being underwritten by the manufacturer, and the manufacturer has assigned a specific dollar amount to the points needed to qualify the audiologist for the trip. This practice in and of itself is explicitly in violation of the *Ethical Practice Guidelines*. Second, the cost of the "points" is not reflected on the invoice to the audiologist. The points earned may be considered a rebate to the audiologist and may be a violation of the federal Anti-Kickback Statute, making it illegal. Third, this trip is far from modest and is based on hearing aid sales; both are violations of the guidelines. The "Frequently Asked Questions" of the *Ethical Practice Guidelines* further clarifies this position by stating: "the acceptance of such gifts, whether related to previous purchases or future purchases, raises the question of whether the audiologist is, in fact, holding the patient's interests paramount. There can be no link between dispensing or referral patterns and gifts" (p. 119 of this book).

Finally, a salient issue that should be considered with this example is the perception this activity creates in the mind of the patient. What would be the patient's perception if the audiologist were to inform the patient that he or she (the audiologist) was receiving a credit towards a Mediterranean cruise because of the hearing aids that were just recommended? According to Hawkins et al (2002), the consumer would most likely view this as a conflict of interest.

Cash Rebates

Hearing instrument manufacturers might offer rebates in the form of cash, gift checks, or some other form of monetary reward, in return for the purchase of a hearing aid or specified number of hearing aids. This is not to be confused with a volume discount, which is reflected on the manufacturer's invoice. Rebates are paid directly to the audiologist, clinic, or facility.

> Scenario 8: The ABC Hearing Aid Corporation announces its Professional Cash Rebate Program. The program details stipulate that for every five ABC hearing aids purchased over the next three months, ABC Hearing Aids will send the audiologist a $150 gift check.

This example bridges several areas that are in violation of the *Ethical Practice Guidelines* adopted by the Academy and ADA: "Incentives or rewards based upon product purchases must not be accepted" (Guideline 1, p. 117 of this book). Gifts or rebates linked to past or future purchases raise the question of whether the audiologist is holding the patient's interests paramount. "There can be no link between dispensing or referral patterns and gifts" ("Frequently Asked Questions," p. 119 of this book). Cash rebates may also violate the federal Anti-Kickback Statutes.

Convention Parties and Dinners

For years audiologists have attended convention parties or dinners that have been underwritten by the various hearing instrument manufacturers. These activities offer an atmosphere in which to socialize with friends, colleagues, and manufacturer representatives. These activities can be beneficial to the collegial atmosphere of the convention. So what could constitute a compromise of ethics or a conflict of interest with the attendance at these parties?

> Scenario 9: The XYZ Hearing Aid Company sends an invitation to attend their convention party on the exclusive scenic harbor cruise. This is an invitation-only event and therefore requires you to RSVP.

Guideline 1 of the *Ethical Practice Guidelines* states: "Audiologists should not participate in any industry-sponsored social function that may appear to bias professional judgment or practice. This would include accepting invitations to private convention parties, golf outings or accepting such items as theater tickets. Meals and social functions that are part of a legitimate educational program are acceptable. When social events occur in conjunction with educational meetings, the educational component must be the primary objective with the meal/social function ancillary to it" (p. 117 of this book). The above convention party scenario was by invitation only, hence a "private" event, which is contrary to the guideline. The cost of the event is not modest and could be construed as a "gift" to preferred accounts. The invitation should therefore be declined.

CONCLUSIONS

Conflict of interest decisions are sometimes clear, with a correct and incorrect path. However, these decisions often fall into gray areas, where cogent arguments can be advanced for differing positions. When confronted with a potential ethical issue regarding a conflict of interest, an audiologist may want to abide by the following suggestions: (1) carefully review the *Ethical Practice Guidelines* (Appendix 1) to determine applicability to the specific situation, and (2) if the situation is not covered, or is not similar to those described in the guidelines or in this chapter, apply the "reasonable person" rule, that is, would a person presented with the facts of the situation reasonably conclude that the audiologist is working in the best interest of the patient? Any amount of skepticism or doubt should help the audiologist avoid placing him- or herself in a position that is a potential conflict of interest. In addition, an Academy member can ask the EPB for an opinion about any particular situation or arrangement.

Audiologists always have the option of not working with manufacturers who offer questionable incentives. If a sufficient number of audiologists employed such an approach, market pressures could lead to more professional relationships between manufacturers and the audiology dispensing community. In the final analysis, however, it is the *audiologist's* responsibility to practice in a manner consistent with the Academy *COE*.

REFERENCES

American Medical Association. (2004) Overview. http://www.ama-assn.org/ama/pub/category/4002.html.

American Medical Association. Council on Ethical and Judicial Affairs. (2004) Gifts to physicians from industry and clarification [Opinion 8.061]. In: *Code of Medical Ethics: Current Opinions with Annotations, 2004–2005 Edition*. AMA Press, 203–214.

Decker TN. (1999) Ethics: conflict of interest in professional practice. *Audiol Today* 11(4):28–29.

Hawkins D, Hamill T, Van Vliet D, Freeman BA. (2002) Potential conflicts of interest as viewed by the audiologist and the hearing-impaired consumer. *Audiol Today* 14(5):27–33.

Chapter 5

Ethics of Professional Communication
Michael J. Metz, Ph.D.

In professional communication—those things spoken or written or otherwise expressed to patients during the course of clinical services—there is a distinct need for ethical considerations. Inevitably, patients interpret the advice of healthcare professionals by making inferences and drawing their own conclusions. But how many times does it turn out that what was said was not what the patient believes was said, or that a patient took meaning from those things that went unsaid? In addition, what is said is oftentimes not as important as the way in which it is said. In certain situations, a person can say nothing at all and yet communicate many things.

Appearance, manner, confidence, and knowledge are certainly important in professional communication. Consider a nonaudiologist dispensing practice that requires medical smocks for every hearing aid dispenser in the office. Further, each salesperson carries a small otoscope in the pocket that is difficult for any customer to miss. Is it the intention of this dress code to imply to the dispenser's customers a level of care that is beyond the scope of the dispenser's license? If these patients subsequently refer to the "nice doctors" who helped with ear molds, or batteries, or warranty repairs, is there fault with the dispenser? Is it enough that the dispensers did not explicitly refer to themselves as "doctors"? Does this office intentionally imply something other than the truth? "Who was hurt?" you might ask. Perhaps a better question would be "Who was served?" It behooves all clinicians to maintain a professional demeanor in every clinical situation; however, it may also serve well to inspect what is implied when communicating with patients.

The goal of this chapter is to pose some situations involving communications that may warrant inspection with regard to their ethical implications. There is sometimes a fine line between communications that are adequate and necessary and those that are nonstandard practice and may be considered ethical violations.

SHARED RESPONSIBILITY FOR PATIENT CARE

Who must share responsibility for patient management and communication? All clinicians recognize that the entire office staff is responsible for what happens in any given office. That is, even though the "ultimate" responsibility lies with the professional, the office staff functions in the clinical setting as an extended health-care team. Given this, the staff is responsible for maintaining operations and performing established protocols, although, ultimately, the responsibility for staff rests on the professional as per Principle 2, Rule 2d, of the American Academy of Audiology (Academy) *Code of Ethics* (*COE*; pp. xv–xxi of this book).

How do you assure that your staff is efficient yet professional? We are constantly reminded of the importance of front office staff in setting the tone for long-term patient relationships. Not only is a friendly face and pleasant demeanor important for a receptionist or the person answering the phone, it is also important that these staff take care not to misrepresent a clinician. Rule 6a of the Academy *COE* states: "Individuals shall not misrepresent their educational degrees, training, credentials, or competence." This misrepresentation is likely not blatant but may be as subtle as the statement by a scheduler that the audiologist is "busy in the hospital," perhaps implying a level of patient responsibility that is more than an audiology license would typically allow. As audiology moves toward autonomy, seeking the level of authority and patient care the field believes it deserves, care must be taken to educate office staff regarding the position of audiology in the health-care arena. Implications such as those above may suggest more than the office (or clinician) warrants.

SECOND OPINIONS

What are the ethical implications of offering patients a second opinion? Second opinions on diagnosis are less likely to pose ethical problems than amplification recommendations. Since some audiologists consider it a breach of collegial behavior, if not unethical, to "steal" patients, it may be worthwhile to examine the traditions of other professions.

The American Medical Association (American Medical Association, Council on Ethical and Judicial Affairs, 2004b, Opinion 8.041) advises physicians that patients are free to seek second opinions, and the original physician should provide case information to the physician who will serve as a consultant. The second-opinion physician is free to take over responsibility for the patient, as the patient's free choice is considered to be of paramount importance. The American Dental Association position (2005, Section 2.B.1) is similar. The patient should be returned to the care of the original dentist after consultation, unless the patient explicitly expresses a different preference.

The American Academy of Orthopaedic Surgeons' *Second or Additional Medical Opinions in Orthopaedic Surgery* (2002) is very specific in regard to second opinions:

Ethics in Audiology

1. Any illegal action is unethical. For example, it would be illegal as well as unethical for the orthopaedic surgeon providing the second or additional medical opinion to slander the referring physician if the slanderous information is known or can be proven to be false.

2. In accepting a patient for consultation, it is ethical for the consulting orthopaedic surgeon to render an opinion and return the patient to the treating physician for continuing care. The consulting orthopaedic surgeon should communicate with the patient as well as the referring physician about the opinion.

It is unethical for the consulting orthopaedic surgeon to solicit care of the patient. However, at the *sole* discretion of the patient, the patient ethically may choose to terminate his or her relationship with his or her treating physician and then enter into another treatment relationship with the consulting orthopaedic surgeon. It is not unethical for the consulting orthopaedic surgeon to accept the patient under these circumstances, although some orthopaedic surgeons choose not to accept the patient because of their personal view that a conflict of interest situation might be created.

Even though this advice pertains to physicians, it would appear that there are many parallels to the practice of audiology. As audiology seeks limited license practitioner status, it would behoove the profession to consider the standards of other autonomous medical professions. One additional provision of the American Dental Association code of ethics (2005) merits discussion:

Section 2.B.1. Second Opinions. A dentist who has a patient referred by a third party for a "second opinion" regarding a diagnosis or treatment plan recommended by the patient's treating dentist should render the requested second opinion in accordance with this Code of Ethics. In the interest of the patient being afforded quality care, the dentist rendering the second opinion should not have a vested interest in the ensuing recommendation.

This reinforces that the patient's interests are to be held paramount. The professional's self-interest must not be a factor.

Consider two scenarios that pose different challenges in ethically providing second opinions. What constraints are imposed if parents are seeking a second opinion about their child's hearing, and are these same constraints applicable if an adult patient seeks a second opinion on what constitutes the most appropriate form of amplification? Sometimes patients shop for different clinical opinions, sometimes for better prices.

In an effort to increase business in a practice, it may not be unusual for a clinician to welcome the chance to offer a second opinion. Sometimes this clinician may try to convince the patient that he or she should remain in that office for clinical care rather than return to the first office. Sometimes the second audiologist is more vociferous than necessary in disagreeing with the first clinician's opinions or findings. Seldom is there a protocol for managing these second opinion patients since, historically, audiology has not discussed this issue. Still, as patients seek treatment for their hearing loss, care should be taken to avoid unethical methods of unfairly diverting patients from the original audiologist's practice.

If the second opinion involves the administration or interpretation of audiologic procedures, the office issuing the second opinion should exercise care in the type of advice given to the patient or the referral source. If the test results and interpretation differ significantly from that obtained from the first clinician, the audiologist offering the second opinion should remember that the differences could arise from factors other than error by the first audiologist. Care should be taken to avoid denigrating the fellow professional. When two professional opinions conflict, other ethical and professional responsibilities arise, including the need for communication between audiologists, consideration of the level of competence of one or both clinicians, and the future benefit to patients yet to be seen by either clinician.

In many situations, it could likely be assumed that the patient would not be seeking the second opinion if he or she were satisfied with the first provider or opinion. Although there are a number of reasons a patient might seek a second opinion, it could be argued that a very common reason for seeking another audiologist's advice would be pricing of prosthetics, services, or procedures.

If the reason for seeking a second opinion involves money, then the ethical issue becomes one of placing the interests of the patient in a primary position, while putting the financial interests of the practice in a secondary position. After all, this view is consistent with all ethical principles that require the patient's interests to be placed in the primary position. In this case, if the usual and customary price of the second-opinion practice is lower, the patient is free to exercise his or her freedom of choice. An ethical issue may arise if the second opinion audiologist were to deliberately undercut the price quoted by the first provider, citing a lower amount than would have been quoted otherwise. That behavior is not consistent with the highest levels of professionalism. It is unlikely that the good of the patient is the clinician's first priority. Similarly, if the patient sought the second opinion for the purpose of clarifying a clinical issue or opinion but the second audiologist interprets the visit as an attempt to find the best price and offers amplification and associated services at a lower cost, then the best interests of the patient may be at risk, constituting unethical behavior on the part of the audiologist. It would seem reasonable to expect that, if a patient truly sought a second opinion regarding a clinical issue, the audiologist would confine the discussion to the clinical issue under consideration. If, however, the patient sought differences in pricing of, say, a hearing aid, then the circumstances no longer involve a clinical opinion but, rather, a financial consideration. The second-opinion audiologist must evaluate the reason for the patient request and act accordingly. If the patient seeks a professional opinion on the accuracy of the diagnosis, then that should be the limit of the opinion provided; however, if the patient is in search of competitive pricing information, then it is ethical to honor that request. If the interests of the patient are always placed in a primary position, then the resulting information or pricing discussion will likely be appropriate.

DISMISSING PATIENTS

Freedom of choice applies not only to the patient but also to the medical provider. The American Medical Association (American Medical Association, Council on Ethical and Judicial Affairs, 2004a, Opinion 9.06) holds that a physician is free to accept or decline an individual as a patient. Similarly, the *Code of Medical Ethics and Professionalism for Orthopaedic Surgeons* states (American Academy of Orthopaedic Surgeons, 2004):

I. C. The orthopaedic surgeon may choose whom he or she will serve. An orthopaedic surgeon should render services to the best of his or her ability. Having undertaken the care of a patient, the orthopaedic surgeon may not neglect that person. Unless discharged by the patient, the orthopaedic surgeon may discontinue services only after giving adequate notice to the patient so that the patient can secure alternative care.

Within the confines of Rule 1a of the Academy *COE* ("Individuals shall not limit the delivery of professional services on any basis that is unjustifiable or irrelevant to the need for the potential benefit from such services"), audiologists also have the freedom to choose the patients for whom they will care, and whom they will dismiss from their care. However, the commonly accepted practice of bundling long-term follow-up with the price of the hearing aid creates issues of contract law. The audiologist would be well advised to communicate with an attorney before dismissing a hearing aid patient who has prepaid for hearing aid care.

In general, patients are dismissed from professional evaluation or treatment for essentially two reasons: either the clinician has completed the course of evaluation or treatment, or the clinician believes that the patient can make better clinical progress with a different approach or provider. The primary interests of the patient being paramount, some patients can also be quite difficult from a cooperation or personality standpoint. So, on occasion, a clinician may consider denying further services to a patient. Underlying this issue is the clinician's responsibility for continuing patient care, and the question of professional ethics in such dismissals.

With particular regard to providing rehabilitative therapy for hearing loss, Rule 5b of the Academy *COE* states: "Individuals may make a statement of prognosis, but shall not guarantee results, mislead, or misinform persons served." As an example, consider the patient who continually returns to a provider's office with complaints of hearing aids that do not function as the patient expects. In this type of situation, it may not be uncommon for the patient to demand services, treatments, or considerations that the provider is unwilling or unable to provide. In the case of a belligerent, overly demanding patient, what might be the factors that would allow the clinician to dismiss this patient from care? Thoughts (and thresholds of action by the clinician) will probably vary on this issue. But paramount to any decision to dismiss a patient from care should be the best interests of the patient. For example, if an audiologist were employed in a public school setting, an uncooperative student cannot be easily dismissed. If a patient in almost any clinical setting continually has problems performing tasks required in the course of diagnostic testing or therapeutic methods, an astute and thorough clinician would search for alternative tests or methods of collecting the needed evaluative data or providing the rehabilitative care. Specifically, if a patient has trouble with his or her hearing aids, clinical competency would require that each problem be adequately investigated and data be accumulated that would support dismissal.

In all clinical situations, the threshold for patient dismissal should be based upon objective data. In a recent discussion of patient dismissal, the American Speech-Language-Hearing Association (ASHA) argues that

> It is the clinician's ethical responsibility to review and analyze all aspects of past services in order to identify specific modification(s) that have the greatest probability of yielding improved outcomes and then implement those improvements with ongoing monitoring. [2004]

The most important concept to be taken from the ASHA statement is the implication that clinical outcomes data serve to determine if a patient can be dismissed from therapeutic care. It is conceivable that personality conflicts or patient belligerence would prevent the patient/clinician relationship from producing therapeutic gain. But a reasonable clinician would likely determine methods of circumventing such conflicts before they reach a critical stage.

According to Tetrault (2002), a clinician can generally dismiss a patient under most circumstances if he or she:

- Gives the patient adequate notice in writing (certified mail, return notice requested) at least thirty days prior to dismissal;
- Provides a brief description of why he or she is terminating the relationship;
- Documents the notification and reasons in his or her records; and
- Offers to provide copies of the patient's records upon receipt of a signed authorization to do so.

See Figure 1 for a sample letter notifying a patient of his or her dismissal from a professional office. In the interests of full disclosure to the patient, as per Rule 5a of the Academy *COE* ("Individuals shall provide persons served with the information a reasonable person would want to know about the nature and possible effects of services rendered, or products provided or research being conducted"), this example letter should in no way be treated as a form letter but merely taken as a suggestion of the manner in which a patient could be notified of dismissal. Adherence to Rule 5e ("Individuals

Audiology Practice
1234 Main Street
Anywhere, VA 12345

[date]

Dear [Patient],

In the course of professional evaluation or treatment, there comes a time when the progress of the patient can no longer be anticipated.

It is my professional judgment that this office can no longer continue to manage your hearing care needs. We believe that significant clinical progress will not result from our continued care of your hearing problems.

If you would like copies of your clinical files for your own or future reference, we would be pleased to provide you with all files in your clinical chart. Please notify our office in the event that you wish to obtain this information, or if you wish it sent to another health-care provider.

Thank you for trusting this office with your hearing care needs in the past. We hope that your experiences with us have been satisfactory.

Sincerely,

[Signature]

Figure 1. Sample letter dismissing a patient.

shall maintain documentation of professional services rendered") should also be considered when preparing such a document, and the dismissing clinician must be able to adequately document the reasons for the dismissal. (The reader is advised to have such a dismissal letter reviewed by an attorney to assure that all legal requirements are met.)

If the audiologist-patient relationship has arisen from contractual services to a hospital, health-maintenance organization, or other provider of managed health care, the audiologist will be bound to the provisions of the contract for services. Generally, these provider contracts, contracts with other payors, as well as some state laws, do not allow "patient dumping." "Patient dumping" is a term that is used to describe the illegal procedure of transferring medically unstable or unwanted patients to other facilities or providers for other than medical (professional) reasons. The term is generally used when hospitals move or refuse patients for financial reasons (Health Care Financing Administration, 1998), but it could also be construed to mean dismissing patients for belligerence, noncooperation, or personality conflicts.

PATIENT ACCESS TO THEIR OWN INFORMATION

State law may govern patient access to health-care information. A general medical tradition is that the clinician owns the medical records but that, upon patient request, copies of those records or a summary must be provided. The professional may institute a nominal charge for providing these copies.

It is difficult to imagine the circumstances under which a health-care provider would not allow a patient access to all pertinent information in his or her own chart; however, there may be some circumstances in which release of certain information would not foster good patient-provider relationships. Consider the situation that involves opinions or conclusions that reflect negatively on the patient. For example, during the course of providing hearing rehabilitation, the audiologist may note that the patient's expectations were out of line with reality, so much so that that patient will likely never attain the outcome the patient wishes. Perhaps the clinician noted the patient's belligerence in some task, or properly charted other negative aspects of the patient's behavior. Full disclosure of the clinician's opinions to the patient may sometimes be difficult or embarrassing.

To withhold any information contained in the patient's chart may not be in keeping with the expected standards of care. Failure to allow access to all information in the patient's chart may be cause for ethical or legal investigations. Perhaps the best solution is to exercise care in the charting of any and all information, forming opinions and conclusions based solely on data and not conjecture.

Two major issues are addressed in this patient access discussion. The first involves the type of charting that is required in any diagnostic or therapeutic encounter. Complete and concise chart notes are necessary if subsequent chart inspection is to demonstrate a true therapeutic plan and outcome (perhaps necessary for insurance or other third-party reimbursement). To imply to the patient and the third party that a therapeutic course was followed and to not chart such a course is considered contrary to the typical standard of practice. Therefore, every clinician is advised to maintain complete and fully descriptive chart notes. To do less may be to provide less than the standard degree of care and thus pose an ethical violation.

The second issue involves the patient's right to access *all* of his or her own data. The law may require such access. But does the patient deserve access to the records that contain payment history from third parties, costs of prosthetic devices, and charges for all types of professional services? Many audiology practices routinely put such information in patient charts. The argument that retail businesses do not disclose wholesale costs would seem to be inappropriately referenced when a health-care provider incorporates this information into the medical record.

How audiologists disclose financial information about hearing aid purchases to patients may impact how others view our profession. If the itemized cost of the hearing aid is not included within the patient chart and is thus not available to the patient under full disclosure policies, the audiologist may be seen as withholding patient information. On the other hand, disclosing all financial information involved in the treatment of a patient is certainly not within the scope of professional care and therefore not subject to the full access requirement placed on other clinical information. It is to be expected that there will be many different methods of handling this access to information, or lack thereof, but there appears to be no generally accepted opinions.

UNBUNDLING AND COMMUNICATION

When dealing with reimbursable diagnostic services, most clinicians in most fields itemize all costs, especially when bills are submitted to third-party payors. However, in audiology, the costs of hearing aids are seldom itemized, or "unbundled." In fact, even the term "unbundling" appears to be a semantically loaded word in that its use causes considerable debate among those audiologists who dispense hearing aids. In general, "unbundling" is a hearing aid term. As noted, diagnostic procedures are almost always itemized.

How is unbundling—or "itemization," if that term is less troublesome—related to communication with patients? Perhaps it is not so much what is said as what goes unsaid. It is currently common practice to manage the purchase of a hearing aid in a "bundled" fashion (all costs for goods and services combined into one price). This is true no matter where or from whom the hearing aid is purchased—audiologist, hearing aid dispenser, or physician. The "bundled" practice is generally thought to have arisen from the retail hearing aid sales model that was the standard of hearing instrument specialists. Since the early specialists were not trained clinicians, and since hearing instruments were not classified in the medical arena until recently, this retail model was the only delivery method.

Unbundling hearing aid device cost and service costs has some advantages relative to patient communication. Releasing the entirety of the medical file, including information on device costs, is no longer uncomfortable. It also permits full and complete patient communication. Itemization does the following:

1. Assigns a separate cost to goods;
2. Assigns a cost, even if only in a relative manner, to all services;
3. Lists the services that would most often comprise the standard of clinical practice; and
4. Assures that listed services were rendered if they have been submitted for payment.

Communication with the patient is served in that the patient is made aware of the exact procedures and their associated costs. If the procedure has value, that value and the associated cost are documented in the billing. Itemization or line-item billing allows for all patients to understand the value of rehabilitative services, including the audiologist's time and knowledge. Indeed, itemization may be the best method for communicating the value of professional services to the patient. A further advantage to unbundling relates to the previously discussed issue of dismissing a patient. The value of services already rendered, and those that will not be rendered to a hearing aid patient who is dismissed, is more easily delineated.

SUMMARY

Communicating with patients involves a great deal more than merely talking to them. Not only do patients misconstrue things said in a clinical situation, but there may be many other nonverbal clues that influence a patient's perceptions. From the procedures and methods of the "front office" staff to the presentation of a billing statement, the maintenance of professional standards reflects on the ethical precepts of all audiologists. Care must be taken to avoid even the occasional miscommunication or unjustified implication.

Finally, perhaps there are some audiologists who think that adherence to a code of behavior similar to that of the medical and dental professions may not be necessary. However, there would likely be negative consequences to relaxing the *Code of Ethics*. Professional ethical codes have evolved over time through attempts to assure the patient that his or her best interests are being upheld by the clinician. Whether borne of the need to assure the patient, the third-party payor, or other members of the profession, a professional code of ethics is essential in any profession. To set ethical goals that reflect only the least common denominator of the profession may do a large disservice to the future of the profession. Taking on the responsibilities of an autonomous profession is a step toward becoming an autonomous profession.

REFERENCES

American Academy of Orthopaedic Surgeons. (2002) *Second or Additional Medical Opinions in Orthopaedic Surgery*. Rev. ed. http://www.aaos.org/wordhtml/papers/ethics/1200eth.htm.

American Academy of Orthopaedic Surgeons. (2004) *Code of Medical Ethics and Professionalism for Orthopaedic Surgeons*. Rev. ed. http://www.aaos.org/wordhtml/papers/ethics/code.htm.

American Dental Association. (2005) *ADA Principles of Ethics and Code of Professional Conduct*. http://www.ada.org/prof/prac/law/code/ada_code.pdf.

American Medical Association. Council on Ethical and Judicial Affairs. (2004a) Free choice [Opinion 9.06]. In: *Code of Medical Ethics: Current Opinions with Annotations, 2004–2005 Edition*. AMA Press, 268–269.

American Medical Association. Council on Ethical and Judicial Affairs. (2004b) Second opinions [Opinion 8.041]. In: *Code of Medical Ethics: Current Opinions with Annotations, 2004–2005 Edition*. AMA Press, 190.

American Speech-Language-Hearing Association. (2004) Admission/discharge criteria in speech-language pathology. *ASHA Leader* Suppl. 24 (April 27):65–70.

Health Care Financing Administration. (1998) Site Review Guidelines. *Federal Register* 63(113).

Tetrault J. (2002) How to dismiss problem patients: balance their demands with your rights. *Physicians Practice* (July–August). http://www.shands.org/professional/ppd/practice_article.asp?ID=145.

Chapter 6

Child and Elder Abuse
Therese C. Walden, Au.D.

All health-care providers are morally and legally responsible for the care of their patients. Included in this responsibility is the ability to recognize the signs of abuse and neglect and the ability to appropriately refer cases to those who can intervene on behalf of the patient. This chapter describes the signs of abuse that audiologists must remain vigilant for, and the course of action to take when a child or elder shows signs of abuse. Also described are the agencies and organizations responsible for the investigation and protection of the child or elder in cases of abuse.

CHILD ABUSE

Most physically abused children never come to the attention of authorities. Neglected children and those who have been sexually abused may have no outward physical signs of harm and are especially hard to identify. The impact of child abuse and neglect is associated with immediate as well as long-term consequences that may include brain damage, developmental delays, learning disorders, problems forming relationships, aggressive behavior, and depression. Survivors of child abuse and neglect may be at greater risk for problems later in life, such as low academic achievement, drug use, teen pregnancy, and criminal behavior. These lasting effects influence not just the child and family but the whole of society (U.S. Department of Health and Human Services, Administration for Children and Families, 2004, p. 5).

Hundreds of millions of dollars are spent annually for infants and children with residual morbidity as a result of abuse and neglect. These expenditures include direct medical care costs as a result of abuse and neglect; federal, state, and local funding used by child protective agencies in preventative and investigative efforts; and foster care expenses for children removed from their homes due to child abuse and neglect.

What Is Child Abuse and Neglect?

Each state is responsible for providing its own definitions of child abuse and neglect that meet federal minimum standards found in the federal Child Abuse Prevention and Treatment Act (CAPTA), 42 U.S.C.A. §5106g, as amended most recently by the Keeping Children and Families Safe Act of 2003. Generally, "child abuse" is a term referring to any recent act or failure to act on the part of a parent or caretaker that results in death, physical or emotional harm, sexual abuse or exploitation, or presents an imminent risk of serious harm. "Sexual abuse" is defined as activities by a parent or caretaker such as fondling, incest, penetration, or indecent exposure. Sexual abuse includes exploitation through prostitution or enticement or coercion to participate in the production of pornographic materials. Neglect is failure to provide for a child's basic needs such as food, shelter, or medical care. Failure to educate a child or attend to special education needs, and inattention to a child's emotional needs or exposure to domestic violence are also considered neglect (U.S. Department of Health and Human Services, Administration for Children and Families, 2004, p. 7).

Who Is Abused?

Children aged birth to three years had the highest rate of abuse, girls slightly higher than boys. According to the U.S. Department of Health and Human Services Administration for Children and Families' report *Child Maltreatment, 2002* (2002), of the 896,000 children found to have been victims of abuse or neglect in 2002, more than half of child victims experienced neglect; almost 20 percent were physically abused; and almost 20 percent were sexually abused or emotionally or psychologically maltreated. Other types of abuse (abandonment, threats of harm to the child, and congenital drug addiction) were also reported. Many children were victims of multiple types of maltreatment. Approximately 1,400 children died in 2002 as a result of child abuse or neglect.

What Are the Warning Signs (Physical and Behavioral) of Child Abuse?

Recognizing the signs of child abuse and neglect is the first step in helping abused or neglected children. A solitary sign of abuse in isolation does not prove abuse is occurring; however, repeated evidence of a specific sign in isolation or a combination of signs warrants a closer look at the circumstances. There are physical as well as behavioral indicators of a child at risk for neglect, abuse, and other forms of maltreatment (Table 1).

Who Are the Abusers?

The overwhelming majority, approximately 80 percent of physical abuse and neglect perpetrators, are parents, acting alone or together. Other relatives, unmarried partners, and persons with other relationships to the child, for example, school employee, camp counselor, and so on, account for the

	Physical Indicators	Behavioral Indicators		Physical Indicators	Behavioral Indicators
Physical Abuse	• Unexplained bruises (in various stages of healing) • Unexplained burns, especially cigarette burns or immersion burns • Unexplained fractures, lacerations or abrasions • Swollen areas • Evidence of delayed or inappropriate treatment for injuries	• Self destructive • Withdrawn and/or aggressive—behavioral extremes • Arrives at school early or stays late as if afraid to be at home • Chronic runaway (adolescents) • Complains of soreness or moves uncomfortably • Wears clothing inappropriate to weather, to cover body • Bizarre explanation of injuries • Wary of adult contact • Apprehensive when other children cry	Sexual Abuse*	• Torn, stained or bloody underclothing • Pain, swelling or itching in genital area • Difficulty walking or sitting • Bruises or bleeding in genital area • Venereal disease • Frequent urinary or yeast infections	• Withdrawn, chronic depression • Excessive seductiveness • Role reversal, overly concerned for siblings • Poor self-esteem, self-devaluation, lack of confidence • Peer problems, lack of involvement • Massive weight change • Suicide attempts (specially adolescents) • Hysteria, lack of emotional control • Inappropriate sex play or premature understanding of sex • Threatened by physical contact, closeness • Unwilling to change clothes in front of anyone • Exhibits fantasy or baby-like behavior • Frequent nightmares • High level of unexplained anxiety
Physical Neglect	• Abandonment • Unattended medical needs • Consistent lack of supervision • Consistent hunger; inappropriate dress, poor hygiene • Lice, distended stomach, emaciated • Inadequate nutrition	• Regularly displays fatigue or listlessness, falls asleep in class • Steals food, begs from classmates • Reports that no caregiver is at home • Frequently absent or tardy • Self destructive • School dropout (adolescents) • Extreme loneliness and need for affection	Emotional Abuse**	• Speech disorders • Delayed physical development • Substance abuse • Ulcers, asthma, severe allergies	• Habit disorder (sucking, rocking, biting) • Antisocial, destructive • Neurotic traits (sleep disorders, inhibition of play) • Passive and aggressive—behavioral extremes • Delinquent behavior (especially adolescents) • Developmentally delayed

* Sexual abuse may be non-touching: obscene language; pornography, exposure—or touching: fondling, molesting, oral sex and intercourse.

** Emotional abuse may be name-calling, insults, put-downs, etc., or it may be terrorization, isolation, humiliation, rejection, corruption and ignoring.

Reprinted with permission from the National Children's Advocacy Center Web site (http://www.nationalcac.org/).

remaining percentage. Women are most frequently the perpetrators and are mostly mothers younger than 40 years old; the male counterparts are typically the children's fathers. The majority of perpetrators in sexual abuse cases are nonrelatives or in a non-child-rearing role. Less than three percent of sexual abuse perpetrators were parents (U.S. Department of Health and Human Services, Administration for Children and Families, 2002).

Who Is Responsible for Reporting Child Abuse?

Reporting suspected child abuse and neglect is everyone's ethical responsibility. However, state laws also impose a legal obligation on certain persons, called "mandatory reporters," to report suspected child abuse or neglect. If there is suspicion or concern about the treatment of a child, a report should be made to the appropriate authorities in the state in which the child resides.

All 50 states, the District of Columbia, and the U.S. territories have enacted statutes specifying procedures that a mandatory reporter (categories described below) must follow when making a report of child abuse or neglect (National Clearinghouse on Child Abuse and Neglect Information, 2003a). Mandatory reporters are individuals who are required by law to report cases of suspected child abuse or neglect. In most states, the statutes require mandatory reporters to make a report immediately upon gaining their knowledge or suspicion of abusive or neglectful situations. In all jurisdictions, the initial report may be made orally to either the child protective services agency or to a law enforcement agency.

Individuals typically designated as mandatory reporters have frequent contact with children. Such individuals include:

- Health-care workers (nurses, allied health professionals, physicians)
- School personnel
- Child-care providers
- Social workers
- Law enforcement officers
- Mental health professionals
- Clergy

More than one-half of reporters of child abuse and neglect are professionals such as educators, medical personnel, child day-care providers, foster care providers, and law enforcement and legal personnel.

All states have a system to receive and respond to reports of suspected child abuse and neglect. If any of the mandatory reporters suspects a child is being harmed, concerns should be reported to the appropriate authorities, such as child protective services. Each state has trained professionals who can evaluate the situation and determine whether intervention and services are needed. Most states have a toll-free number to call to report suspected child abuse and neglect.

How to Report Abuse and Neglect

For information on how and where to file a report of suspected child abuse and neglect, contact the Childhelp USA® National Child Abuse Hotline. Professional crisis counselors can be reached 7 days a week, 24 hours a day, at the Childhelp USA® toll-free number: 1-800-4-A-CHILD (1-800-422-4453) (National Clearinghouse on Child Abuse and Neglect Information, n.d.). The counselor will help direct the reporting individual to the most appropriate agency. First reporting varies by state; for example, if the alleged abuser is a family member or caregiver, then the abuse is reported to the state's child protective services agency. If the alleged abuser is not someone responsible for the child, then the call is placed to 911 for emergency services. If you, the audiologist, are the first person to receive such information from a child, or if you suspect abuse is occurring, you are legally responsible to report the alleged abuse.

Exceptions to and Limitations of Patient Confidentiality

In terms of patient confidentiality (an ethical issue) and privacy (a legal issue), the audiologist is protected under state and federal statutes when reporting suspected abuse or when reporting alleged abuse conveyed to the audiologist directly by the child. Also, it is not the responsibility of any mandatory reporter to investigate the abuse prior to reporting to the appropriate agency (Center for School Mental Health Assistance, 2003).

Child Protective Services (CPS)—Child Welfare Systems

The nation's child welfare system gives states the responsibility and the authority to intervene in situations where a child is, or appears to be, in need of protection as a result of abuse or neglect. In the United States, state CPS agencies receive more than 50,000 allegations of child abuse or neglect each week. On average, two-thirds of these cases will meet federal and state policy for conducting an assessment or investigation. After interviewing or meeting with family members, the alleged victim, and others associated with the case, the CPS agency makes a decision as to whether the child was a victim of abuse, neglect, or other form of maltreatment.

Child protective services agencies provide preventative as well as postinvestigation services to victims of child abuse and neglect. Preventative services are provided to help parents and other caregivers increase their understanding of child rearing and child development through the use of parenting education, housing assistance, day-care services, substance abuse treatment, and other educative processes. Post-investigation (remedial) services are offered on a voluntary basis or as ordered by the courts to ensure the child's safety. These services may include individual counseling, foster care, family-based and court services.

The Office on Child Abuse and Neglect (OCAN), a division of the Children's Bureau, Administration for Children and Families, U.S. Department of Health and Human Services (HHS), takes the federal lead in the effort to educate individuals and communities on how to prevent child abuse and neglect. Generally, child abuse and neglect prevention activities focus on four main areas (U.S. Department of Health and Human Services, Administration for Children and Families, 2002):

- Creating and distributing public awareness material and information;
- Developing and using skills-based curricula to teach children to recognize and resist child abuse;
- Conducting parent education and parent support programs; and
- Providing home visitation programs for families at risk.

Federal and State Regulations/Laws

Child abuse and neglect are defined in both federal and state legislation. The Federal Child Abuse Prevention and Treatment Act (CAPTA) provides the foundation on which state definitions are based. CAPTA established a minimum set of standards that define child maltreatment. Each state is then responsible for its own definitions of child abuse and neglect that meet these standards within its civil and criminal codes. In order to receive federal grant money, CAPTA requires states to approve legislation that provides for immunity from prosecution arising out of the reporting of abuse or neglect. All 50 states, the District of Columbia, and the U.S. territories have laws that provide some form of immunity from criminal and civil liability for persons who report suspected child abuse or neglect in "good faith" (National Clearinghouse on Child Abuse and Neglect Information, 2003b). State licensing boards can require training in child abuse recognition and intervention prior to initial licensure or license renewal for all mandatory reporters.

The National Clearinghouse on Child Abuse and Neglect Information, a service of the Children's Bureau, maintains an online searchable database and publishes summary documents related to select state child abuse and neglect, child welfare, and domestic violence laws. This database is not intended to take the place of appropriate legal counsel.

Under the Health Insurance Portability and Accountability Act (HIPAA) of 1996 and the Privacy Rule of the U.S. Department of Health and Human Services, the protected health information for patients is subject to federally mandated standards for use and disclosure. A covered entity (health-care provider) is permitted to disclose protected health information, without the patient's authorization, for the purpose of reporting child abuse or neglect (45 C.F.R.§164.512[b][ii]). This disclosure is allowed such that the use of the protected health information maintains a balance between the privacy of the patient and the safety and protection of the patient (U.S. Department of Health and Human Services, Office for Civil Rights, 2003).

Internet Resources for Information on Child Abuse

- http://nccanch.acf.hhs.gov/
  National Clearinghouse on Child Abuse and Neglect Information (a service of the Children's Bureau)

- http://nccanch.acf.hhs.gov/general/legal/
  National Clearinghouse on Child Abuse and Neglect Information
  (state mandates)

- http://nccanch.acf.hhs.gov/pubs/factsheets/about.cfm
  Child Abuse Prevention and Treatment Act (federal legislation)

- http://www.acf.dhhs.gov/acf_services.html#caan
  U.S. Department of Health and Human Services—Services for Families,
  Child Abuse and Neglect

- http://www.jimhopper.com/abstats/
  Jim Hopper's personal Web site—Child Abuse: Statistics, Research, and
  Resources

- http://www.nationalcac.org/
  The National Children's Advocacy Center (NCAC) is a nonprofit agency
  providing prevention, intervention, and treatment services to physically
  and sexually abused children and their families within a child-focused
  team approach. Since opening in 1985 as the nation's first Children's
  Advocacy Center, the NCAC has become a leader in the field of prevention
  and intervention of child maltreatment. To contact: 210 Pratt Avenue,
  Huntsville, AL 35801; Phone: 256-533-5437; Fax: 256-534-6883.

ELDER ABUSE

Elder abuse is a societal problem that continues to gain recognition worldwide. Both the United Nations Economic Council and the World Health Organization have launched initiatives to increase awareness of elder abuse as a human rights issue. Policymakers and practitioners have sought ways to protect older Americans from physical, psychological, and financial abuse for more than 40 years. It is difficult to say how many elders are abused, neglected, or exploited, in large part because inspection is limited and the problem remains greatly hidden. While a couple of studies place the estimate of elder abuse, neglect, and exploitation at 4–6%, other estimates are even higher (Alliance for Aging Research, 2003). One consistent finding, over a ten-year study period, is that reports of elder abuse have increased each year, perhaps owing to increased awareness of the problem and the availability of viable options in terms of intervention (National Center on Elder Abuse, 2003a).

What Is Elder Abuse?

"Elder abuse" is a term referring to any knowing, intentional, or negligent act by a caregiver or any other person that causes harm or a serious risk of harm to a vulnerable adult. Elder abuse can affect people of any ethnic background or social status and can affect both men and women. The specificity of laws varies from state to state, but broadly defined, abuse may be (National Center on Elder Abuse, 2003b):

- Physical Abuse—Inflicting, or threatening to inflict, physical pain or injury on a vulnerable elder, or depriving him or her of a basic need.
- Emotional Abuse—Inflicting mental pain, anguish, or distress on an elder person through verbal or nonverbal acts.
- Sexual Abuse—Nonconsensual sexual contact of any kind.
- Neglect—Refusal or failure by those responsible to provide food, shelter, health care, or protection for a vulnerable elder.
- Abandonment—The desertion of a vulnerable elder by anyone who has assumed the responsibility for care or custody of that person.
- Financial or Material Exploitation—The illegal or improper use of an elder's funds, property, or assets.

What Is Self-Neglect?

Self-neglect is characterized as the behavior of an elderly person that threatens his or her own health or safety. Self-neglect generally manifests itself in an older person as a refusal or failure to provide himself or herself with adequate food, water, clothing, shelter, personal hygiene, medication (when indicated), and safety precautions. The definition of self-neglect excludes a situation in which a mentally competent older person, who understands the consequences of his or her decisions, makes a conscious and voluntary decision to engage in acts that threaten his or her health or safety as a matter of personal choice. Signs and symptoms of self-neglect may include dehydration, malnutrition, untreated medical conditions, and poor personal hygiene; unsafe living conditions; unsanitary living areas, manifested by something such as a nonfunctioning toilet; inadequate clothing and lack of the necessary medical aids such as eyeglasses, hearing aids, and dentures; and grossly inadequate housing or homelessness (National Center on Elder Abuse, 2003b).

Who Is Abused?

Each year hundreds of thousands of older persons are abused, neglected, and exploited by family members and others. Many victims are people who are older, frail, vulnerable, and depend on others to meet their most basic needs (Administration on Aging, 2004). Social isolation and mental impairment (such as dementia or Alzheimer's disease) are two factors that may make an older person more vulnerable to abuse. But in some situations, studies show that living with someone else (a caregiver or a friend) may increase the chances for abuse to occur. A history of domestic violence may also make a senior more susceptible to abuse.

What Are the Warning Signs or Risk Factors of Elder Abuse?

While one sign alone may not be indicative of a problem, health-care providers should be alert to the following (National Center on Elder Abuse, 2003b):
- Bruises, pressure marks, broken bones, abrasions, and burns may be an indication of physical abuse, neglect, or mistreatment.
- Unexplained withdrawal from normal activities, a sudden change in alertness, and unusual depression may be indicators of emotional abuse.

- Bruises around the breasts or genital area can occur from sexual abuse.
- Sudden changes in financial situations may be the result of exploitation.
- Bedsores, unattended medical needs, poor hygiene, and unusual weight loss are indicators of possible neglect.
- Behavior such as belittling, threats, and other uses of power and control by spouses are indicators of verbal or emotional abuse.
- Strained or tense relationships and frequent arguments between the caregiver and elderly person are also signs.

Who Are the Abusers?

Abusers of older adults are both women and men. Family members are more often the abusers than any other group. For several years, data showed that adult children were the most common abusers of family members; recent information indicates spouses are the most common perpetrators when state data concerning elders and vulnerable adults are combined. As far as the types of abuse are concerned, neglect is the most common type of abuse identified (National Center on Elder Abuse, 2003b).

Who Is Responsible for Reporting Elder Abuse and Self-Neglect?

Everyone has an ethical responsibility to keep vulnerable elders safe from harm. However, there are two general categories of reporters. A permissive reporter is any person, such as someone who works for a bank, an attorney, or volunteers in a facility or program providing services for vulnerable adults. Mandatory reporters are professionals identified by state law who must make a report if they have reason to believe that the abuse, abandonment, neglect, or financial exploitation of a vulnerable adult has occurred. Mandatory reporters depend on the particular state's law but may include (National Center on Elder Abuse, 2003b):

- Law enforcement personnel
- Social workers
- Professional school personnel
- Contracted individual providers
- Employees of a social service, welfare, mental health, home care, hospice, home health, adult day care, and adult day health agency
- Owners or employees of nursing homes, boarding homes, or adult family homes
- Health-care providers (physicians, nurses, allied health professionals)

Reporting Elder Abuse or Neglect

If there is suspicion that an elder is in immediate, life-threatening danger, call 911 or the local police. If the danger is not immediate but there is a suspicion that abuse has occurred or is occurring, report this information to the state or local adult protective services agency. (This may be the state APS unit, the county department of social services, or an agency on aging.) If the elder is a nursing home resident, call the state long-term care ombudsman. If you are not sure whom to call, contact the nationwide toll-free Eldercare Locator number (1-800-677-1116) (http://www.eldercare.gov/), and they will refer you to the appropriate state or local agency. Although it is the legal and ethical responsibility of all health-care professionals to report suspected abuse, it is recommended that the adult patient be informed before the reporting takes place. As an adult, the patient's autonomy and self-governance takes precedence, and even though the reporter tries to keep paramount the patient's welfare and safety, the patient can request that the health-care professional not intervene.

Adult Protective Services

Adult protective services (APS) agencies are located in each state, and the APS office should be contacted to report suspected elder abuse or self-neglect. The National Elder Abuse Center Web site lists hotline numbers for each state at http://www.elderabusecenter.org/. The APS agency receives and screens reports of elder abuse for potential seriousness, and calls are confidential. If the agency decides the situation possibly violates state elder abuse laws, it assigns a caseworker to conduct an investigation. In emergency cases, a caseworker can be assigned more quickly, usually within 24 hours. If the victim needs crisis intervention, services are available. If elder abuse is not substantiated but self-neglect or basic living or medical care services are needed, the APS agency will work as necessary with other community agencies to obtain those services. The elder has the right to refuse services offered by APS. The APS agency provides services only if the senior agrees or, as a last resort, has been declared incapacitated by the court and a guardian has been appointed (Administration on Aging, 2004).

Federal and State Regulations/Laws

The Older Americans Act Amendments of 2000 was signed into law on November 13, 2000. The act provides for funding of state programs to prevent elder abuse under subchapter III, "Grants for State and Community Programs on Aging."

Legislatures in all 50 states and the District of Columbia have passed some form of elder abuse prevention laws. Laws and definitions of terms vary considerably from one state to another, but all states have set up reporting systems (Center for Social Gerontology, n.d.). If an audiologist suspects or becomes aware of elder abuse, then that audiologist should report the suspected abuse to the appropriate authorities. Most states have laws that would make the audiologist, or any reporter, exempt from retaliation if the report was made in good faith and if the circumstances of the report of suspected abuse are such that a reasonable person would conclude similarly. No person can be held liable, civilly or criminally, if they report in good faith.

Under the Health Insurance Portability and Accountability Act (HIPAA) of 1996 and the Privacy Rule of the U.S. Department of Health and Human Services, protected health information for patients is subject to federally mandated standards for use and disclosure. A covered entity (health-care provider) is permitted to disclose protected health information, without the patient's authorization, about an individual that the covered entity "reasonably believes" is a victim of abuse, neglect, or domestic violence, provided that (a) the individual whose protected health information is disclosed agrees to the disclosure; (b) the disclosure is required by law; or (c) the disclosure is authorized by law and the covered entity believes disclosure is necessary to prevent serious harm to the individual or others (45 C.F.R. § 164.512[c]). In most cases, the covered entity must promptly inform the individual of the disclosure. This disclosure is allowed such that the use of the protected health information maintains a balance between the privacy of the patient and the safety and protection of the patient (U.S. Department of Health and Human Services, Office for Civil Rights, 2003).

Internet Resources for Information on Elder Abuse

- http://www.elderabusecenter.org/
  National Center on Elder Abuse (NCEA): The NCEA is administered by the National Association of State Units on Aging as the lead agency and funded by grant No. 90-AP-2144 from the U.S. Administration on Aging.

- http://tcsg.org/
  The Center for Social Gerontology (TCSG): The TCSG is a "non-profit research, training and social policy organization dedicated to promoting the individual autonomy of older persons and advancing their well-being in society." At this Web site there are links to legal services providers for older Americans, listed by state.

- http://www.elderabusecenter.org/default.cfm?p=statehotlines.cfm
  Adult Protective Services (APS): APS protects vulnerable adults by investigating allegations of abuse, neglect, abandonment, and financial exploitation. To report elder abuse, contact APS through your state's hotline. Toll-free numbers provided at the NCEA Web site.

- http://www.aoa.gov/eldfam/Elder_Rights/Elder_Abuse/Elder_Abuse.asp
  Administration on Aging (AOA), Department of Health and Human Services: This site provides an outline of a wide range of topics, programs and services related to aging. The AOA provides home and community-based services to millions of older persons, funded under the Older Americans Act.

REFERENCES

Administration on Aging. (2004) Elder abuse. http://www.aoa.gov/eldfam/Elder_Rights/Elder_Abuse/Elder_Abuse.asp.

Alliance for Aging Research. (2003) Get mad . . . respect your elders. *Living Longer and Loving It!* 15(Winter). http://www.agingresearch.org/living_longer/winter_03/elders.cfm.

Center for School Mental Health Assistance. (2003) *Child Abuse and Neglect Reporting Procedures.* http://csmha.umaryland.edu/resources.html/resource_packets/download_files/child_abuse_report_2003.pdf.

Center for Social Gerontology. (N.d.) Law and aging. State legal services development. Listing of state legal services providers for older americans: by state. http://tcsg.org/.

National Center on Elder Abuse. (2003a) Abuse statistics. http://www.elderabusecenter.org/default.cfm?p=abusestatistics.cfm.

National Center on Elder Abuse. (2003b) Frequently asked questions. http://www.elderabusecenter.org/default.cfm?p=faqs.cfm.

National Clearinghouse on Child Abuse and Neglect Information. (2003a) *Reporting Laws: Immunity for Reporters.* State Statutes Series 2003. http://nccanch.acf.hhs.gov/general/legal/statutes/immunity.cfm.

National Clearinghouse on Child Abuse and Neglect Information. (2003b) *Reporting Procedures.* State Statutes Series 2003. http://nccanch.acf.hhs.gov/general/legal/statutes/repproc.cfm.

National Clearinghouse on Child Abuse and Neglect Information. (N.d.) Resources for reporting child abuse and neglect. http://nccanch.acf.hhs.gov/topics/reporting/guidelines.cfm.

U.S. Department of Health and Human Services. Administration for Children and Families. (2002) *Child Maltreatment, 2002.* Department of Health and Human Services. http://www.acf.hhs.gov/programs/cb/pubs/cm02/index.htm.

U.S. Department of Health and Human Services. Administration for Children and Families. (2004) *Gateways to Prevention: What Everyone Can Do to Prevent Child Abuse. 2004 Child Abuse Prevention Community Resource Packet.* 2nd ed. http://nccanch.acf.hhs.gov/topics/prevention/order/packet2004.pdf.

U.S. Department of Health and Human Services. Office for Civil Rights. (2003) *Summary of the HIPAA Privacy Rule.* http://www.hhs.gov/ocr/privacysummary.pdf.

Chapter 7

Ethical Issues in Practice Management

Debra Abel, Au.D.
Robert Hahn, J.D.

"Beneficence" is repeatedly mentioned in ethics literature and is highly applicable to audiology. "Beneficence" is defined as "acting in the interests of the patients." Its counterpart is "nonmaleficence," which means "do no harm" (Jonsen et al, 1998). These are the hallmarks of any health-care profession and are the benchmarks to which the profession should adhere. It is the intent of this chapter to address the daily, and also the unusual, scenarios with which we may be confronted in our own facilities while keeping the above tenets in the forefront in our clinical practice. These scenarios raise issues that run the gamut from confidentiality to treatment of patients, the release of information, supervision, and billing practices, to name a few.

CONFIDENTIALITY

Principle 3 of the *Code of Ethics of the American Academy of Audiology* (*COE*; see pp. xv–xxi of this book) states: "Members shall maintain the confidentiality of the information and records of those receiving services or involved in research." With the enactment of the Health Insurance Portability and Accountability Act (HIPAA), breach of patient confidentiality may also violate the law. HIPAA was enacted in 1996 as Public Law 104-191 "to improve portability and continuity of health insurance coverage in the group and individual markets, to combat waste, fraud and abuse in health insurance and health care delivery, … to simplify the administration of health insurance, and for other purposes." According to HIPAA privacy regulations, when treatment, payment, or operational (TPO) information is needed, the patient's written authorization is not required. However, in a litigious society, it is prudent to obtain one for any exchange of information, in order to protect your patients, your practice, and yourself.

Authorization in the form of written consent for a specific event or time frame is required for purposes other than health-care treatment, payment, or operations. For example, audiologists need permission from parents to confer with school personnel regarding school-aged patients who wear amplification and are in need of FM capability. A sample authorization form is included in Figure 1. You may prefer to devise your own, which must include specific elements. The form should include the name and address of your practice or facility, and the patient's name, address, and birth date. In addition, the information that needs to be released or that will be released by you to a third party, with his or her identifying information, should be included, as well as an expiration date. The patient's right to revoke the authorization also needs to be addressed, as well as a notification that the information may be redisclosed by the recipient.

The HIPAA privacy rule requires that disclosures of patient information, even of TPO, be kept to the minimum of information necessary. Also, we need to keep uppermost in our minds, when speaking with colleagues, that we do not reveal the name of the patient in the interesting clinical case we may be describing. This is not considered treatment, payment, or operations information. If recounting a case in a presentation or journal article, the name has to be redacted and any identifying information deleted, unless the patient has authorized the disclosure of such information.

The HIPAA privacy rule went into effect on April 14, 2003. Therefore, every practice should already have a HIPAA compliance program and be in compliance. The HIPAA privacy regulation is very complex and detailed, and this discussion is only intended as a broad overview.

STARK LAW

There are a variety of federal and state laws designed to prevent health-care fraud. These laws are intended to protect patients from substandard care, and to protect health-care programs, such as Medicare and Medicaid, from abuse (Medicare and Medicaid Web site: http://www.cms.hhs.gov). This chapter will discuss two of the most important federal antifraud laws: the Stark Law and the federal Anti-Kickback Statute. Many states also have their own state Stark laws and/or state anti-kickback laws, but such state antifraud laws are beyond the scope of this chapter.

All audiologists should be aware of the federal antifraud laws as well as any relevant state antifraud laws. Before embarking on a previously uncharted contractual arrangement with a physician or physician group, an audiologist should consult legal counsel familiar with health-care fraud and abuse laws. The Stark Law and the Anti-Kickback Statute should be considered separately; activities or arrangements that are acceptable under one may violate the other.

John F. Smith, Au.D.
123 Medical Way
Smalltown, VA 12345
703-555-1234
Fax 703-555-5678

Release of Information

I,_____ (___/___/_____), authorize the
            Patient's name   Birth date

release of my _____
                          Desired health information

from ___/_____/_____ to ___/_____/_____ to be released to:
       Date   Date

_____
          Practice name

_____
          Practice address

This authorization expires one year from the date above. This authorization
may be revoked in writing at my request. I understand charges for
duplicating my records may be incurred.

_____
          Patient's name

_____
          Patient's address

_____

Witnessed by: _____

Date: _____/_____/_____

Figure 1. Sample form authorizing release of information.

The Stark Law (42 U.S.C. § 1395nn) prohibits physician "self-referrals."[1] That is, it prohibits a physician (or a physician's immediate family member) from referring patients for designated health services to an entity in which the physician (or his or her immediate family member) has a financial relationship, unless a specific exception applies. The law also prohibits the entity receiving the prohibited referral from billing for those designated health services.

The Stark Law is a civil, not a criminal, law. Violations may result in denial of reimbursement, mandatory refunds of federal payments, civil money penalties, and exclusion from federal and state health-care programs. The Centers for Medicare and Medicaid Services (CMS) has issued regulations (42 C.F.R. Part 411) implementing the Stark Law in two phases over a period of several years, and there may yet be a third phase.

Let us look at the elements of a Stark Law violation. To violate Stark, there must be a *referral* by a physician (or his or her immediate family member) to an *entity* in which the physician (or his or her immediate family member) has a *financial interest* for the furnishing of *designated health services* (DHSs). A "referral" is any physician request for, order of, or certification or recertification of the need for DHS to be paid under Medicare. If the referring physician personally performs the service, there is no referral. A referral by an audiologist is not covered by Stark, unless the referral is directed or controlled by a physician. An "entity" is any person (including an individual, partnership, or corporation) who furnishes DHS. A person is considered to be furnishing DHS if it is the person to which CMS makes payment or to whom the right of payment has been reassigned. Thus, an audiologist may be an entity receiving a prohibited referral. A "financial interest" is broadly defined to include a direct or indirect ownership or investment interest or a direct or indirect compensation arrangement. "Designated health services" (DHSs) are defined as the following items and services only:

- Clinical lab services;
- Physical therapy, occupational therapy, and speech-language pathology services;
- Radiology and certain other imaging services;
- Radiation therapy services and supplies;
- Durable medical equipment and supplies;
- Parenteral and enteral nutrients, equipment, and supplies;
- Prosthetics, orthotics, and prosthetic devices and supplies;
- Home health services;
- Outpatient prescription drugs; and
- Inpatient and outpatient hospital services.

Because of this narrow definition of DHS, the Stark Law has limited application to audiologists. Services provided in a hospital, both inpatient and outpatient, are one category of audiology services that fall within the definition of DHS. However, since the entity furnishing DHS is the entity that receives payment from CMS, and since CMS reimburses the hospital for inpatient and outpatient services, it is the hospital (not the audiologist) that must comply with the Stark Law. Two other eligible services are the Current Procedural Terminology (CPT) codes 92507 and 92508 (treatment of speech, language, voice, communication or auditory processing; individual and group, respectively). CMS considers these procedures to be speech-language pathology services, and therefore DHS. Because DHS must be payable by Medicare, these procedures are DHS when furnished by an audiologist "incident to" a physician's services. However, even if an audiologist were to perform these services pursuant to a prohibited referral, they would in most cases be exempt from the Stark Law under the "in-office ancillary services" exception. Audiology diagnostic tests, including cochlear implant mapping and reprogramming (CPT codes 92601 through 92604), are not DHS. In addition, CMS has clarified that hearing aids are not DHS.

The Stark Law and implementing CMS regulations provide a number of exceptions. These include bona fide employment relationships, arm's-length agreements for the rental of office space or equipment, and "in-office ancillary services." To qualify for an exception, a transaction or arrangement must meet specific requirements. For example, to qualify for the in-office ancillary services exception, the services must meet a supervision requirement (e.g., furnished by an individual under the supervision of the referring physician), a building requirement (e.g., furnished in the same building in which the referring physician normally furnishes services to patients), and a billing requirement (e.g., billed by the supervising physician, the group practice, an entity wholly owned by the physician or group practice, or an independent third-party billing company acting as agent of the physician, group practice, or entity). Because the Stark Law has limited impact on audiologists, we will not discuss the roughly 30 exceptions in detail in this chapter.

In summary, the Stark Law prohibits a physician (or his or her immediate family member) from referring a patient for the furnishing of DHS to an entity in which the physician (or his or her immediate family member) has a financial interest, unless an exception applies. The Stark Law does not significantly affect audiologists because it only applies to referrals for the furnishing of DHS, and because the only audiology services that are DHS are inpatient and outpatient hospital services and CPT codes 92507 and 92508. In the case of hospital services, CMS makes payment to the hospital, so the hospital is the entity that must comply with Stark. In the case of CPT 92507 and 92508, in most situations these services would fall under the exception for "in-office ancillary services." Audiologists should be aware, however, that most states have their own Stark laws, and some of these may be broader than the federal Stark Law. Whenever in doubt, audiologists are advised to consult legal counsel well versed in federal and state Stark laws.

ANTI-KICKBACK STATUTE

The federal Anti-Kickback Statute (AKS) (42 U.S.C. § 1320a-7b) addresses the offering, giving, soliciting, or receiving of kickbacks in return for referrals of patients whose items or services are reimbursable under federal health-care programs. It prohibits any person from "knowingly and willfully solicit[ing] or receiv[ing] any remuneration (including any kickback, bribe, or rebate) directly or indirectly, overtly or covertly, in cash or in kind," to induce someone to refer an individual for "any item or service for which payment may be made in whole or in part under a Federal health care program" (except the Federal Employees Health Benefits Program [FEHBP]). The AKS prohibits kickbacks because (1) they create an incentive to overutilize reimbursable services, increasing costs to Medicare and other federal health-care programs; (2) they distort medical decision making; and (3) they result in unfair competition by freezing out qualified providers who are unwilling to pay kickbacks.

The AKS is a criminal statute. Violation of the AKS is a felony punishable by imprisonment, heavy fines, or exclusion from federal health-care program participation. Unlike the Stark Law, which is a civil law, intent is a critical element that must be proved by the prosecutor. However, while intent to induce referrals or obtain money for referrals must be proven, it is not required to be the only purpose of the remuneration. The AKS is enforced by the Office of Inspector General (OIG), not CMS.

The elements of an AKS violation are the following:

- Intent: acting knowingly and willfully.
- Offering, giving, soliciting, or receiving remuneration.
- Referral of patients who purchase, lease, order, or arrange to receive any item or service reimbursable under a federal health-care program, except FEHBP.

The AKS is much broader than the Stark Law. Unlike Stark, it is not limited to particular designated health services. Instead, it applies to any item or service payable in whole or in part under any federal health-care program other then FEHBP. A number of possible arrangements between audiologists and physicians may implicate the AKS. Here are a few examples:

- An audiologist furnishes diagnostic tests to a physician's patients at no or reduced charge in return for hearing aid referrals, where hearing aids are covered by the state Medicaid plan. The audiologist is giving the physician remuneration (i.e., free or reduced price diagnostic tests) in return for referrals of hearing aid business reimbursable by Medicaid.
- An audiologist rents office space from a physician and pays rental based on the number of referrals of Medicare/Medicaid

patients received from the physician. The audiologist is giving the physician remuneration (i.e., above-market rent) in return for referrals of Medicare/Medicaid business.

- An audiologist accepts remuneration (in the form of gifts, entertainment, loans, cooperative marketing funds, or other benefits) from a hearing aid manufacturer in return for prescribing the manufacturer's hearing aids, where the hearing aids are covered by Medicaid or another federal program (other than FEHBP). The audiologist is receiving remuneration in return for recommending purchase of hearing aids reimbursable by Medicaid.

To avoid criminalizing innocent conduct, there are a number of "safe harbors" to the AKS. If a transaction meets all the requirements of a safe harbor, it is protected from prosecution. However, failure to qualify for a safe harbor does not automatically mean a transaction is in violation of the AKS. The safe harbors include (1) arm's-length agreements for the rental of office space or equipment, (2) discounts, and (3) bona fide employment relationships. While a complete discussion of the AKS safe harbors is beyond the scope of this chapter, two of the safe harbors are worth mentioning because of their widespread use.

To qualify for safe harbor protection, a discount must be "a reduction in the amount a buyer (who buys either directly or through a wholesaler or a group purchasing organization) is charged for an item or service based on an arms-length transaction" (42 C.F.R. § 1001.952[h][5]). The discount must be made at the time of sale (or, if a rebate, the terms of the rebate must be fixed and disclosed in writing to the buyer at the time of sale). The buyer receiving the discount must, upon request of the OIG or state regulators, provide certain information provided to it by the seller. In addition, the discount must be properly disclosed and reflected in the charges billed to the federal health-care program paying for the item or service. Thus, the discount must benefit the Medicare or Medicaid program. The discount also must be earned in the same fiscal year as the purchase of the applicable item or service. The safe harbor does not protect discounts in the form of cash payments (or cash equivalents).

The *Ethical Practice Guidelines on Financial Incentives from Hearing Instrument Manufacturers* position statement of the American Academy of Audiology (Academy) and the Academy of Dispensing Audiologists (ADA) (see Appendix 1) educates the members of these organizations about the ethics and legality of the acceptance of trips, cash, and other gifts in exchange for recommending items that may be paid for by a federal health-care program. Abiding by these guidelines protects the audiologist from inadvertent violations of the Anti-Kickback Statute. We recommend that all audiologists read and adhere to these guidelines.

To qualify for the office rental safe harbor, an audiologist must ensure that rental payments are not disguised kickbacks to induce referrals by the physician-landlord:

- The rental agreement must be in writing and signed by the parties;
- The rental agreement must cover all premises rented by the parties and specify the premises;
- The term of the agreement must be at least one year;
- If the audiologist is renting space for periodic intervals, the agreement must specify the exact schedule of usage;
- The aggregate rental amount must be set in advance, consistent with fair market value, and may not take into account the volume or value of referrals; and
- The aggregate space rented may not exceed what is reasonably necessary to accomplish a commercially reasonable business purpose.

For a more detailed discussion of this safe harbor, see the OIG *Special Fraud Alert: Rental of Space in Physician Offices by Persons or Entities to Which Physicians Refer* (Office of Inspector General, 2000).

Many states have their own anti-kickback laws, which may differ from the federal AKS. Whenever in doubt, legal counsel well versed in both federal and state anti-kickback laws should be consulted.

INFORMED CONSENT

Some patients do not seek audiological treatment under their own volition, but by that of a well-meaning relative or friend. The patient has the ultimate right of determining treatment. When patients are incapacitated and unable to make their own decisions, it is recommended that a power of attorney act on their behalf. It is suggested that the patient's signature on your practice registration form be obtained, indicating that the patient is granting permission to provide the necessary audiologic diagnosis and treatment options. For those 18 years or younger, a note from the parent or guardian is necessary in order to provide audiologic services in that parent or guardian's absence.

BILLING PRACTICES

The Academy *COE* states in Rule 4b: "individuals shall not charge for services not rendered." In order to be reimbursed for the work performed, it is necessary to abide by absolute standards when billing third-party payors.

When billing payors who reimburse invoice costs for hearing aid purchases, the actual invoice is the one to be submitted, not one that inflates the price. By the same token, the invoice must reflect all discounts. Not providing the actual invoice is fraudulent, and the audiologist may be subject to prosecution. This prosecution may lead to the revocation of state license, to say nothing of a potential prison sentence, fines, and the payback of any monies obtained under fraudulent conditions.

The audiologist needs to consult the signed insurance contract in addition to the explanation of benefits to determine if balance billing is allowed. "Balance billing" is having the patient pay for whatever their insurance company or companies may not have paid on their behalf for the services rendered. Many insurance companies will allow balance billing on the hearing aid invoice, but not on the dispensing fee. Balance billing a patient incorrectly may lead to the termination of that insurance contract, and the audiologist may be required to return any fees incorrectly billed to the patient or the insurance company. Each insurance company will have different benefits, so the audiologist needs to be familiar with each contract.

The mechanism for assigning a code for the patient's diagnosis is by using the ICD-9-CM codes. Utilizing "signs and symptoms" or the clinical findings/outcomes/processes is accepted practice. Any inaccurate portrayals or misrepresentations are fraudulent, even if the audiologist has the altruistic intention to provide the patient with better reimbursement. Upcoding may also be considered fraudulent and should not be attempted. "Upcoding" is billing a higher-level or more complex code than the procedure performed in order to receive a higher level of reimbursement. An example would be billing a higher level of an evaluation and management (E & M) code than the levels of service and time actually performed. Medicare will not reimburse audiologists for these codes, but other third-party payors may. Unbundled billing of the separate components of 92553, 92555, and 92556 instead of the bundled 92557 code is considered illegal practice, as is charging for testing not performed. The audiologist needs to be aquainted with modifiers that are appended to a CPT code to reflect such things as performing air conduction unilaterally as it is considered a bilateral code. That modifier would be "-52" in this example.

Itemization, or unbundling, is a current "hot topic" in audiology and relates to how hearing aids and services are billed. Many third-party payors (such as the United AutoWorkers' contracts) require that the hearing aid acquisition fee and the dispensing fee be delineated, charged, and coded separately. Many audiologists have been doing this for some time and also charge for conformity evaluations or rechecks when a patient returns for hearing aid related services. (Again, check the contract and the Explanation of Benefits [EOB] to know what the patients' and the audiologist's responsibilities entail). In the instances where insurance coverage is not involved, the practice may bundle or unbundle as appropriate according to the business philosophy, state insurance laws, and what the community will support.

Providing services at a greater frequency or for an extended period of time when no reasonable expectation for patient benefit exists (such as vestibular rehabilitation or tinnitus treatment) is not ethical practice and may constitute insurance fraud (Abel and Hamill, 2004). By the same token, hearing aids should not be dispensed when success cannot be attained or be reasonably expected.

DOCUMENTATION

Documentation is critical for accountability. The *COE* in Rule 5e states: "individuals shall maintain documentation of professional services rendered." If any additional reports need to be submitted to a third-party payor, these must be accessed readily. Chart notes need to provide detailed information of patient complaints and symptoms, interpretation for procedures performed, recommendations or impressions, phone calls, and so forth made on the patient's behalf. Chart entries need to be dated and signed. Other critical information includes patient history, pertinent family history, and medications. The documentation needs to support the billing code used and should be such that if someone unfamiliar with this patient were to provide services to that patient, it is clear what has been done, why, and what is indicated for further diagnosis or treatment.

A generally accepted guideline is this: " 'If I can't code your encounter form from your documentation, then your documentation is inadequate.' In fact, disputes over payments will be settled by looking at the documentation, not the encounter form" (K. Dennis, email message to D. Abel, 2003). In other words, if it is not documented, it did not happen.

REFERRING TO ANOTHER AUDIOLOGIST

Principle 2 of the *COE* states: "Members shall maintain high standards of professional competence in rendering services." Rule 2a prescribes that "members shall provide only those professional services for which they are qualified by education and experience." Rule 2b elaborates, "Individuals shall use available resources, including referrals to other specialists, and shall not accept benefits or items of personal value for receiving or making referrals."

With expansion of the scope of practice of audiology, some audiologists may not be proficient in all areas. Some audiologists have become specialists with cochlear implants, vestibular diagnosis and rehabilitation, neurophysiologic measurements, tinnitus management, and the like. If an audiologist is unable to competently provide services, he or she must refer the patient to a qualified colleague. The patient will appreciate the audiologist's integrity in recognizing his or her limitations. Proper referral lessens your liability and better serves the patient.

DISPARAGING COLLEAGUES

It is not professional to criticize another audiologist to a patient when it appears the other audiologist did not perform to the standards of the profession. A patient may have misinterpreted what was said or been confused, or there may be other sides to the story. If there is a question of an ethical violation on the part of that audiologist, according to Rule 8c of the Academy *COE*, that person should be reported to the Chair of the Ethical Practice Board (EPB).

CULTURAL/RELIGIOUS BARRIERS

The *COE* Rule 1b reads "Individuals shall not provide services except in a professional relationship, and shall not discriminate in the provision of services to individuals on the basis of sex, race, religion, national origin, sexual orientation, or general health." If presented with a difficult cultural or religious barrier, the audiologist may need to contact those in the cultural or religious community to inquire about those barriers in order to be respectful of them. Local colleges and universities may offer the needed educational background. They may also be aware of any interpretive services required in order to communicate with the patient in the most effective way.

ACCEPTING GIFTS FROM PATIENTS

Often patients are grateful for the work done and the help given. Token gifts such as candy, food, and books are acceptable. However, cash should not be accepted as a gift and is only to be accepted when a specific billed service has been provided. Garstecki (2000) recommends that gifts from patients should always be directed to work teams or organizations, rather than to individual service providers. He also states that it is in the audiologist's best interest not to accept gifts or other considerations that may give the appearance of affecting professional judgment or integrity.

DISCLOSURE OF A CONFLICT OF INTEREST TO PATIENTS

Any monetary or special interests that the audiologist may have with a manufacturer should be disclosed to the patient. This may be done within the practice's marketing material or by disclosing privately to the patient. For example, if the audiologist were a field trainer for a particular manufacturer (EZ Fit-EZ Money), and that patient were to be fit with an EZ Fit-EZ Money instrument, in counseling, the audiologist would tell the patient that familiarity with the device comes both from dispensing the product and working as a manufacturer's trainer who teaches other hearing health-care practitioners about the product. The audiologist may continue to explain that the manufacturer pays for the training services but that the work has no effect on the practice's account. The clinical rapport developed with that patient could be undermined if he or she discovered that the audiologist had a financial relationship with the manufacturer of their instruments and did not disclose it. By providing the disclosure, the patient is free to seek a second opinion if concerned about the audiologist's objectivity.

IMPAIRED PRACTITIONERS

Rule 8b states, "individuals shall not engage in dishonesty or illegal conduct that adversely reflects on the profession." With the stressful lives we lead, there is the danger of being an impaired practitioner, whether drug or alcohol induced. If suffering from drug or alcohol abuse, whether the drug is legal or not, the audiologist and patient are placed at risk. The personal and professional liability is not worth the cost. Audiologists who know of a colleague who is impaired have several options. Intervention strategies with friends and families can be of help if you are not comfortable discussing this with them on a one-on-one basis. Intervention is used to make the impaired practitioner aware of his or her problem and suggest ways to combat it. Audiologists have the ethical burden to report their colleague to the EPB for review, and state licensure laws may compel you to report your suspicions about the licensee to that board as well.

INCOMPETENT PATIENTS

Principle 4 of the *COE* states, "Members shall provide only services and products that are in the best interest of those served." Rule 4a specifies, "individuals shall not exploit persons in the delivery of professional services." Audiologists often serve the elderly, some of whom may be confused or forgetful. In many instances, these patients are unaware that they are experiencing these symptoms. Dementia may be accompanied by belligerence. Such a patient will require specialized care. If you cannot provide this care, refer him or her to a colleague who can. Working closely with the family of this challenging patient may help you select the most appropriate care; for example, an assistive listening device may be recommended instead of a hearing aid.

TRAINING/CONTINUING EDUCATION

The *COE* Rule 2f states, "Individuals shall maintain professional competence, including participation in continuing education." Professional status resides in the knowledge base, expertise, and skill levels that one acquires through experience and ongoing continuing education. Not providing patients with access to state-of-the-art technology and knowledge is a liability and a violation of the above rule in addition to many state licensure laws. Again, if an audiologist is untrained in performing a specific procedure, he or she should seek the appropriate training before delivering that particular procedure. This may include formal continuing education training or being mentored by a colleague who performs the procedure of interest often and expertly.

MARKETING

Untruthful advertising raises ethical issues and has legal consequences (Panneback et al, 1996). One issue relates to guaranteeing results of clinical intervention or benefit from products dispensed. An audiologist can legitimately make such claims only when they can be substantiated by objective and published data. Results from clinical studies employing well-controlled scientific measures and rigorous statistical analyses may be cited in professional advertisements in ways that support the interest of the audiologist and that do not misrepresent the findings or mislead the reader (Garstecki, 2000).

Audiologists shall not represent their training or credentials in any way that would be deemed false or misleading (Rule 6a of the COE). State licensure laws on advertising also need to be reviewed. Those who are employed within an organization may find that there are institutional advertising guidelines.

SELLING OF A PRIVATE PRACTICE

The cooperative payment of advertisements by the audiologist and a manufacturer is not recommended as it forges a potentially unethical alliance. As per the *Ethical Practice Guidelines on Financial Incentives from Hearing Instrument Manufacturers* (Appendix 1), the manufacturer can share in the cost of advertising, but only if it is not in reciprocation for past business and only if there is no agreement to dispense a certain number of that manufacturer's aids as a form of repayment. Similarly, manufacturer support of open houses is permitted, but the audiologist must ascertain that the product dispensed is the one best suited for the patient and is not chosen because of the manufacturer's sponsorship of the open house.

If selling or closing a private practice, patients should be informed within a reasonable amount of time to ensure that they receive uninterrupted audiologic services. This may be accomplished with a letter, newspaper advertisements, Web page notices, or other reasonable means. Some state laws and insurance plans may require a minimum of 30 days prior notice.

PROFESSIONAL OBLIGATIONS

According to the COE's Rule 8c, "individuals shall inform the Ethical Practice Board when there are reasons to believe that a member of the Academy may have violated the Code of Ethics." As difficult and uncomfortable as this may be, in order to be an autonomous and self-regulating profession that is accountable to its members and those whom they serve, any known or reasonably suspected infractions or violations of the Academy COE should be reported to the Chair of the EPB (see the COE, Part 2, "Procedures for the Management of Alleged Violations"). These suspected violations will be investigated, and the accused member will have a fair opportunity to present his or her account of the facts and circumstances.

NOTE

1. The Stark Law is sometimes referred to as "Stark II." The statute originally only prohibited physician referrals to labs in which the referring physician has a financial interest ("Stark I"). When the statute was broadened to prohibit physician referrals to any entity in which the referring physician has a financial interest, it was designated "Stark II."

REFERENCES

Abel D, Hamill T. (2004) Don't "fall" into hazardous practice. *Audiol Today* 16(4):30.

Garstecki D. (2000) Morals, ethics, laws and clinical audiologists. *Semin Hear* 21(1):21–31.

Jonsen A, Siegler M, Winslade W. (1998) *Clinical Ethics: A Practical Approach to Ethical Decisions in Clinical Medicine.* 4th ed. New York: McGraw-Hill.

Office of Inspector General. (2000) *Special Fraud Alert: Rental of Space in Physician Offices by Persons or Entities to Which Physicians Refer.* http://www.oig.hhs.gov/fraud/docs/alertsandbulletins/office%20space.htm.

Panneback M, Middleton GF, Vekovius GT. (1996) *Ethical Practices in Speech-Language Pathology: Case Studies.* San Diego, CA: Singular Publishing Group.

Chapter 8

Ethical Considerations in Supervision of Audiology Students and Employees

Teri Hamill, Ph.D.
Jane M. Kukula, Au.D.

There are ethical considerations when audiologists are called upon to supervise office staff, other professionals, or students. The American Academy of Audiology (Academy) *Code of Ethics* (*COE*; see pp. xv–xxi of this book) has rules applicable to supervision; however, in some cases, ethical decisions cannot be guided by these rules and decisions but, rather, will be decided using a utilitarian approach (see Chapter 3), wherein the chosen course of action creates either the least harm or the greatest benefit. This chapter reviews the rules governing ethical supervision, then discusses some conflicts that are not resolved by applying the *COE*.

THE *CODE OF ETHICS* AS IT RELATES TO SUPERVISION

A profession's code of ethics is a deontological set of rules that binds members of a profession to specific moral conduct. This set of rules addresses relationships between the professional and those in a position of trusting the professional. There are four rules in the *COE* that specifically apply to supervision and support personnel:

- Rule 2d: Individuals shall provide appropriate supervision and assume full responsibility for services delegated to supportive personnel. Individuals shall not delegate any service requiring professional competence to unqualified persons.
- Rule 2e: Individuals shall not permit personnel to engage in any practice that is a violation of the Code of Ethics.
- Rule 4c: Individuals shall not participate in activities that constitute a conflict of professional interest.

- Rule 6b: Individuals' public statements about professional services, products, or research results shall not contain representations or claims that are false, misleading, or deceptive.

Rule 2d states that the supervision must be appropriate in the context of each specific situation. The audiologist must assess the skills of the student or support person, as they relate to the needs of the patient. For instance, a student may have greater experience and skill with adult hearing aid fittings and less with pediatric fittings. Thus, the student is in need of greater supervision and critique when working with a pediatric hearing aid fitting. Because Rule 2d specifically states that services requiring professional competency shall not be delegated to unqualified persons, the audiologist must ensure that students and support persons are properly prepared. Tasks should not be delegated until the audiologist is assured of the competence of the student or support person to perform any given task. Rule 2d further states that the supervisor is responsible for the work performed by support personnel. This also is true for supervision of students. The audiologist must remain accountable, even when not directly providing the service.

Rule 2e applies to all members of the Academy and is especially salient for those in supervisory roles. Preceptors/supervisors can both model ethical conduct and mentor ethical behavior in those supervised.[1] Students are observing all aspects of the externship site; they are exposed to many ethical issues, such as the facility's relationships with manufacturers, billing and coding practices, and hearing aid fitting procedures. The ethical behaviors students are exposed to will influence their future ethical practices, as will be discussed later in this chapter.

Prior to 2003, the *COE* had a rule that read, "individuals shall not accept compensation for supervision or sponsorship beyond reimbursement of expenses." This was rescinded, as it prohibited universities from compensating supervisors in any manner, even preventing preceptors from attending free university-sponsored continuing education events. With this rule deletion, universities and employers may compensate preceptors. However, preceptors must not receive compensation directly from a student. Clearly that would create a conflict that is prohibited by Rule 4c.

Rule 6b asserts that "individual's public statements about professional services, products, or research results shall not contain representations or claims that are false, misleading, or deceptive." Referring to a student or support person as an "audiologist," or allowing a student or support person to use this designator or any other that might give the wrong impression to the patient is misleading. However, use of the term "student audiologist" is permitted.

OTHER CODES OF ETHICS AND LICENSURE REQUIREMENTS

As professionals, there may be several entities that have governing authority, some of which are voluntarily joined and others that have statutory authority. In case of voluntary professional associations, we consent to the organization's authority. The act of joining a professional association requires agreement to abide by its rules, including its code of ethics. Adherence to the rules of an association is compulsory because membership implies to the public a willing acceptance of the publicly declared ethics of the association. Failure to abide by the code of ethics of an association could result, in the extreme cases, in expulsion, with consequential loss of access to member benefits and services, and possible loss of respect of peers and colleagues.

Of even greater concern to the audiologist are rules, regulations, and codes of ethics written into state licensure laws. Egregious violations of state laws can have severe repercussions. Revocation of a license bars a professional from practice in that state; suspension prevents a professional from practicing for a period of time. Even receiving a reprimand may affect the ability to bill third-party payors.

As professionals, we are obliged to adhere to all codes and rules that are mandatory and to which we are willingly subject. Supervisors need to investigate all applicable requirements (both ethical and legal), practice within those boundaries, and ensure that supervisees also adhere to these codes and laws.

IMPORTANCE OF PROPERLY IDENTIFYING STUDENT STATUS

Just as in medicine (American Medical Association, Council on Ethical and Judicial Affairs, 2004a), those receiving audiology services have the right to be informed that a student is providing care, and they have the right to refuse student services. Students should ideally be referred to as "students," and terms that could potentially confuse a patient, such as "Au.D. candidate," should not be used (see further discussion of this issue in Chapter 9).

CONFLICTS ARISING FROM BALANCING STUDENT AND PATIENT NEEDS

The clinician's job is to provide good patient care. Formal education, coupled with years of experience, allows the audiologist to competently handle varied challenges, from effectively counseling patients, to coaxing responses from children, to providing mental tasks for the vestibular patient while evaluating nystagmus. Allowing a student to enter the practice may negatively affect quality of care. By way of example, assume that an Au.D. student begins an externship under the audiologist's supervision and is not fully prepared for the range of clinical skills required in that practice. In the course of the first day, the preceptor is not convinced that the amplification candidate fully understood the value of directional microphones as explained by the student. During a pediatric evaluation, the student's sequence of stimulus presentations during VRA (visual reinforcement audiometry) testing was not optimal; the child lost interest in the task, and the audiometric information is incomplete. During ENG testing (electronystagmography), the student did not give fast, challenging mental tasking; the patient may have suppressed the nystagmus. What should the preceptor do?

A common reaction to this supervisory conundrum is for the preceptor to take over the role of the clinician, relegating the student to observer status. This provides the patient with the best care and can be justified if today's patient is the primary focus. Unfortunately, observation alone seldom improves student performance; students gain from active, more than passive, learning (Rassi, 1987). The next time the student encounters a similar situation, she or he will probably only have marginally better performance. Taking over cannot be the only supervisory strategy in the preceptor's book.

Preceptors on the other end of the spectrum who focus primarily on the need of the student may have the philosophy that it is best to be a "hands-off" supervisor. Such a laissez-faire approach assumes that the student learns best from self-analysis of strengths and weaknesses, and functions better when not made nervous by the preceptor looking over his or her shoulder. Preceptors who deliberately avoid micromanaging the activities of students may reflect on their own personal growth as clinicians as evidence to support this position. The dangers in adopting this approach are myriad. The preceptor may be unaware of problems. Students do not always recognize their shortcomings and ask for needed assistance. The preceptor is legally and ethically responsible for patient welfare. Failure to intervene when necessary to ensure accurate diagnosis and appropriate treatment cannot be justified with the "greater good" theory—that the benefit to future patients outweighs the disadvantages of lower-than-optimal quality of care to current patients.

This book is not intended to be a text in supervision. Our intention is not to detail all the strategies available to maximize student learning while optimizing patient care. We offer general guidelines, however, in the hope that preceptors will consider whether they have had adequate training in supervision to allow them to balance patient care and student training needs.

Supervision theory holds that preceptors should carefully assess student strengths and weaknesses, allowing progressive autonomy. Preceptors should encourage self-evaluation, and assess the accuracy of the self-evaluation, so that preceptors know whether a student can be trusted to seek help when appropriate. Preceptors should be ready to provide concrete, concise instruction, and students should have been prepared to expect this form of direct instruction. Preceptors should be ready to allow students to make and learn from their mistakes when the mistakes can be readily remediated. Appropriate supervision involves creative problem-solving strategies; it is hard (though rewarding) work.

This chapter will next examine some of these concepts as they apply to the case of the ineffective directional-microphone hearing aid counseling described above. Ideally, the preceptor would have evaluated the student's self-perceived abilities before asking the student to counsel a patient. The preceptor could have considered role playing to assess the student's skill level. The preceptor should, and did in this case, observe initial counseling sessions, rather than trusting that the student's advice will be correct and correctly understood. In the scenario suggested here, where the student does not clearly explain the benefits of directional microphones, the preceptor may wish to probe the patient's understanding, which can demonstrate the patient's confusion to the student. "Mrs. Smith, the benefits of directional microphones are hard to understand. Given what you've learned so far, would you help us understand, from your perspective, the advantages and disadvantages of including directional-microphone technology in your hearing aid?" If the student cannot clarify misconceptions, the preceptor should take over as counselor only for that portion of the session, and allow the student to participate in other areas of counseling. Follow-up role playing would allow the student an opportunity to practice counseling and the preceptor an opportunity to evaluate the student's progress.

The vestibular and pediatric testing examples illustrate situations where direct coaching is more advantageous. If the preceptor rapidly switches between modeling the needed strategy and asking the student to emulate the strategy, skill development is better than if the student passively observes. In the pediatric illustration, the preceptor can demonstrate how to properly change stimulus type and pace stimulus presentation, then let the student present the stimuli while the preceptor prompts the next desired action. The preceptor might then tell the student that he or she will now stop the direct instruction to observe the student's next actions, providing guidance only as needed. Similar strategies would assist the student in properly mentally tasking the patient during the ENG testing. Showing the student the return of nystagmus when the patient is tasked correctly would be instructive and reduces the chance that the student dismisses the instruction as "every supervisor just wants things done in their particular way."

While it may sound as if supervision strategies can eliminate the preceptor's conflicts, they do not. It is likely that the preceptor is the better clinician, and if so, relinquishing patient care means that the quality of care decreases. The supervisory process moderates this quality decrease. Preceptors must balance the need to train the next generation and to meet the needs of current patients.

Quality supervision requires dedication, intelligence, and time, but without willing preceptors, the profession cannot continue nor transition to a doctoral-level profession. Preceptors are rewarded with the knowledge that the skills the preceptor has cultivated will benefit the student's numerous future patients. Additionally, preceptors will gain from the process. Students have up-to-date information; they will likely teach the audiologist in some areas. Students can share techniques learned in other clinical rotations that may benefit the practice. The enthusiasm that students bring is reinvigorating. The experience may also allow reflection and renew the preceptor's appreciation of his or her own unique skills.

PRECEPTORS AS GUARDIANS OF THE PROFESSION

Appropriate supervision involves giving students performance feedback. Preceptors enjoy giving encouraging news. Informing the student of deficit areas is harder. What should the preceptor do when the student does not appear to have adequate understanding of the clinical principles? What if the student's knowledge base is inadequate for practice in the current setting? What if the student is not making the expected clinical progress? What if the preceptor cannot justify recommending a passing grade?

Early constructive criticism is key to good supervision and learning. If specific strengths and limitations can be identified, it is possible to construct a remediation plan for the student. The more concrete the feedback, the better the chance that the student can improve to the preceptor's satisfaction. For example, a fourth-year student who requires 45 minutes to conduct a routine adult hearing evaluation obviously requires remediation. Feedback that is limited to global comments may be unhelpful and may have unintended negative consequences. The student may adopt inappropriate shortcuts in order to become time efficient. Feedback that coaches the student to recognize false positive responses that are causing overtesting identifies a problem and permits a concrete solution. Sharing time-saving tricks such as, "Don't put the pen down; keep it in your hand," helps the student tackle efficiency problems directly.

Rarely, the preceptor will encounter a student who is unable to benefit from the given placement, or whose clinical growth is not progressing appropriately. Relegating that student to the few tasks that he or she is able to complete with a reasonable degree of autonomy will not permit the student's skills to improve significantly. The preceptor needs to have open communication with the university faculty to discuss options. However, the preceptor cannot allow external pressure to bias the evaluation of the student. The student's previous performance or progress should not be a consideration in evaluating current performance. While it is possible that the student had progressed appropriately at a previous placement, that does not invalidate the preceptor's perceptions. Joint supervisory evaluation by a faculty member and the preceptor may be appropriate.

The practicing clinician-preceptor has an important role as guardian of the profession. If the student is not performing at an acceptable preprofessional level, the preceptor needs to provide that evaluative judgment, regardless of consequences. Preceptors are responsible for ensuring that they welcome into the ranks of their colleagues those who possess the needed patient-care skills, and that they protect the public by preventing those who are unprepared from practicing independently. This involves careful decision making and introspection regarding whether any personal bias might be affecting professional judgment.

DUAL RELATIONSHIPS IN SUPERVISION OF STUDENTS AND EMPLOYEES

A dual relationship exists if the supervisor has a professional supervisory role and an additional role that may compromise objectivity in the supervisory role (British Psychological Society, 2003). Examples include:

- being a relative of the supervisee;
- supervising either someone who is in a position of authority over you in another context or the close friend or relative of someone in such a position; and
- supervising a close personal friend or lover.

In each case, the additional relationship could create a situation where the supervisor may not be entirely objective. For example, if the department chair seeks dual certification and enrolls as a student, the preceptor could be expected to have difficulty providing critical feedback.

Most frequently, the nature of the dual relationship is that of mentor, confidant, and friend. As social beings, it is not uncommon that preceptors/managers/employers and students/employees develop friendships when they work closely together. There are advantages to workplace friendships. Students can benefit from having a mentor to guide them; they can learn workplace etiquette and values by being fully integrated, including socially, with the staff. Additionally, students and new employees may have recently moved and not have a well-developed supportive social network, and they may look to the preceptor for personal advice.

Workplace friendships between supervisors/employees can aid in maintaining office morale. Humans are social creatures and appreciate friendships within the workplace. However, Yager (n.d.) notes that employees typically seek casual friendships rather than seeking to be "best friends" with other employees, which mitigates the potential deleterious effects of dual relationships.

Dual relationships can be problematic when the unequal power in the relationship is not recognized and appropriately dealt with. Since the supervisor has more power, there is the danger that the supervisor could exploit that power (Bernard and Goodyear, 1992). The supervisee/student may feel uncomfortable declining social invitations or feel unable to resist doing favors for the supervisor. For example, let us say that the supervisor asks the subordinate, "Would you mind picking me up tomorrow? My car is in the shop," or "Could you possibly babysit for me Saturday night?" Can the subordinate decline without feeling that there may be workplace repercussions or ill feelings?

Developing social relationships may also inappropriately erode the authority with which the supervisor is vested. After being granted personal favors, will the supervisor truly be free to objectively evaluate the subordinate and provide critical feedback?

To avoid the potential for the dual relationship to become problematic, certain guidelines should be followed.

- Do not accept supervisory responsibility for close friends, family members, or persons who have authority over you in another capacity.
- Clearly define the limits of the supervisory relationship and the personal relationship. In some cases, direct discussion of the issues may be appropriate. For example, in curtailing gossip or "venting" about another employee, it would be appropriate to explain that as supervisor to both parties, you need to retain objectivity. When accepting a wedding invitation, but declining the bachelorette or bachelor party invitation, you might mention your rationale.
- Avoid acceptance of any gift, from a student or employee, that could raise the appearance of conflict of interest.
- If personal relationships develop, continually evaluate whether there is risk of exploiting the supervisee or of lacking the objectivity necessary to deal impartially and fairly. If either situation is a potential risk, then either the more intimate relationship or the supervisory relationship cannot continue (Bernard and Goodyear, 1992).
- Avoid physical contact. The subordinate may misinterpret the meaning of such gestures in light of the unequal power within the relationship.

Given the comments above, the reader likely anticipates the authors' highly cautionary comments regarding entering into sexual relationships. When there is unequal power, the rule is simple: Don't! A supervisor's overtures can be, and have been, construed as sexual harassment. As is the tradition in other health-care professions, the supervisory relationship should be severed before entering into a personal relationship (American Medical Association, Council on Ethical and Judicial Affairs, 2004b). Beyond fears that the relationship could be coercive given unequal power in the relationship, there is also worry about objectivity. During the relationship, necessary supervisory critical information may not flow; after the end of the relationship, the criticism could be copious, diverse, and some of it may even relate to job function.

SELF-ASSESS SUPERVISORY SKILLS

Being a good clinician does not necessarily equate to being a good supervisor, manager, or preceptor; different skill sets are involved. As discussed above, preceptors need to balance the patient's needs and the student's needs, providing the student with opportunities to learn by doing. Being a preceptor involves careful observation and keen perception of the student's strengths and weaknesses. Similarly, supervision of other professionals and support staff requires the ability to make good observations and accurate judgments. Supervision also requires organizational, interpersonal, and managerial skills that differ from those required of a clinician. If you are newly assuming a supervisory role, it may be appropriate to seek mentoring and to read appropriate literature.

PREPARE APPROPRIATE JOB DESCRIPTIONS AND COMMUNICATE JOB EXPECTATIONS

When interviewing and hiring, be sure that the employee has a copy of the job description. Review the job description when conducting routine employee evaluations to ensure that the description matches the work tasks. This is particularly true in regard to the supervision of support personnel. Over time, clerical staff may change roles as they learn how to handle patient-care needs, such as changing batteries and repairing battery doors, thereby advancing to technician duties. See the Academy's position statement on the audiologist's assistant for information on appropriate task delegation and supervision (American Academy of Audiology, 2006). Licensure laws should also be checked when personnel advance in job capabilities. Registration or licensure may be required of employees who perform certain patient-care tasks.

MODELING PROFESSIONAL BEHAVIOR

Preceptors and supervisors should model professional behavior. Supervision influences professional identity and moral responsibility. Hyrkas and Paunonen-Ilmonen (2001) report that quality of care is influenced by clinical supervision and that ethical awareness and behavior is encouraged through the supervisory process.

Berggren and Severinsson (2003) studied nursing supervisors' methods and means of teaching ethical decision making. They found that supervisors focus on assisting students in deliberating about the case and identifying priorities. The preceptors serve as role models and prioritize patient-care issues and issues of professional autonomy in ethical decision making. They share not only their technical knowledge but also their own values, which allows students to express themselves more freely. Demonstration of moral integrity and responsibility were seen as key components of good supervision.

Given this research, supervisors should be prepared, consider priorities, and structure sessions with students. Preceptors should be accessible and willing to share knowledge, skills, and ethical values. They should share the decision-making process and let students see the process used in prioritizing clinical and supervisory issues. Exposing students to ethical considerations opens the lines of communication for discussion of ethical issues. Preceptors should be a sounding board for students to work through their own ethical dilemmas. They should assist students in the consideration of Beauchamp and Childress's (1994) basic ethical principles of autonomy, beneficence, nonmaleficence, and justice when working through their own ethical issues, and use these same principles in evaluating the treatment of the student (Berggren and Severinsson, 2003). Respect for the student establishes a relationship that recognizes and affirms the supervisee. Students observe the preceptor and are influenced by the supervisor's behaviors and interactions. If a preceptor behaves in an unethical, unprofessional manner, students receive the message that inappropriate behaviors are acceptable.

Open discussions of patient care dilemmas are appropriate. How are difficult situations involving patients or professionals resolved? How are conflicting demands on time and attention handled? How does one assure a complete assessment when there is a waiting room full of patients? Students benefit from discussing these issues. The preceptor may consider establishing office standards of care and explaining their importance to the student.

BILLING ISSUES IN STUDENT SUPERVISION

Preceptors are teachers and must not allow business considerations to inappropriately influence the tasks the student is assigned. The skills of the student, needs of the patient, and requirements of the insurer must all be considered when assigning a task. Professionalism dictates that the preceptor place these needs above financial temptations. "Creative" billing (e.g., unbundling diagnostic services, charging for services not rendered) and conflicts of interest, or even their appearance, must be avoided. Improper maximization of income by inappropriate tasking of students, and unethical billing and coding habits are of special concern. The purpose of an externship is the development of clinical skills leading to independent practice. As students learn and develop, they need, and should be granted, increasing independence. Maintaining appropriate balance between the needs of the patient, the student, and the constraints of applicable rules and laws requires mature thought and action. Preceptors must work with students in order to meet Medicaid and Medicare requirements and should not allow students to have an independent patient load.

Medicare rules have been interpreted as requiring that covered diagnostic services provided by students, and billed to the government, be directly supervised. The most defensible plan would be to provide over-the-shoulder supervision, 100 percent of the time, in these cases (B. Freeman, pers. comm., June 7, 2004).

The recent revision of Medicaid's definition of an audiologist provided clarification on the role of the supervising audiologist. The focus on "treatment" is of course inappropriate, but the general philosophy of the Centers for Medicare and Medicaid Services on supervision is clear. The following is from the *Federal Register*, May 28, 2004:

> We interpret the authority to provide services "under the direction of" an audiologist to mean that a federally qualified audiologist who is directing audiology services must supervise each beneficiary's care. To meet this requirement, the qualified audiologist must see the beneficiary at the beginning of and periodically during treatment, be familiar with the treatment plan as recommended by the referring physician or other licensed practitioner of the healing arts practicing under State law, have continued involvement in the care provided, and review the need for continued services throughout treatment. The supervising audiologist must assume professional responsibility for the services provided under

his or her direction and monitor the need for continued services. The concept of professional responsibility implicitly supports face-to-face contact by the qualified audiologist at least at the beginning of treatment and periodically thereafter. Thus, audiologists must spend as much time as necessary directly supervising services to ensure beneficiaries are receiving services in a safe and efficient manner in accordance with accepted standards of practice. To ensure the availability of adequate supervisory direction, supervising audiologists must ensure that individuals working under their direction have contact information to permit them direct contact with the supervising audiologist as necessary during the course of treatment.

. . . In all cases, documentation must be kept supporting the qualified audiologist's supervision of services and ongoing involvement in the treatment services. Because Medicaid law requires that documentation be kept supporting the provision and proper claiming of services, appropriate documentation of services provided by supervising audiologists, as well as services performed by individuals working under the direction of a qualified audiologist, are necessary. Absent appropriate service documentation, Medicaid payment for services may be denied providers.

Where appropriate, audiology services must adhere to all State requirements and State practice acts governing the provision of services under the direction of a qualified audiologist. As with all Medicaid benefits that permit services furnished under direction, both Federal and State requirements must be met at the time services are furnished for the Medicaid program to appropriately provide Federal financial participation for services furnished on behalf of Medicaid eligible individuals.

Medicaid and Medicare mandates apply only to those covered by these insurance plans; they do not apply to noncovered services, or when other insurers are billed. If the state provisionally licenses the student, billing for services conducted without direct supervision may be permitted (B. Freeman, pers. comm., June 7, 2004); however, this remains a controversial issue.

ASSIGNING APPROPRIATE LEARNING TASKS

As previously mentioned, preceptors should assign tasks based on the abilities of students and support personnel. When a student lacks skill in an area, for example, ENG, keep the student involved. Have the student take the history, give instructions, assist with maneuvering the patient, and so on, and incrementally involve the student in other areas of testing so that she or he develops competence. Avoid the temptation of assigning the student only tasks that he or she has mastered, such as routine audiograms and servicing walk-in patients. The student needs to gain proficiency in advanced procedures. Working jointly with the student can ensure quality care and provide growth experiences for students.

STATE LICENSURE AND OTHER LEGAL ISSUES IN STUDENT SUPERVISION

Knowledge of state licensure laws is necessary for both supervisors and students. Among many things, licensure laws mandate who needs a license, determine scope of practice, affect billing abilities, and have rules applying to supervision of students and possibly support personnel. Penalties for practice outside of state law can be high. In extreme cases, noncompliance can result in revocation of the supervisor's license and lead to the eventual denial of license to a student. Even less severe discipline such as a reprimand can affect reimbursement by third-party payors.

First, a preceptor must pay attention to his or her own credentials. Late renewal of a license has much greater significance than the late renewal of a certificate. If one renews late enough, his or her license can expire. Though practice without a license may legally be a minor offense in most states, billing insurers, especially Medicare, for services while a license is expired is a felony.

Second, state requirements regarding the clinical training of students vary widely. All states require extensive supervised clinical training. Master's-degreed audiologists who perform supervised clinical experience as postgraduates obtain state licensure. Some states require a provisional license for this experience. As the profession moves to a new model of education, requirements for fourth-year Au.D. students are even more varied. Some states accept the students' fourth-year training as equivalent to the supervised experience performed as a postgraduate, and some accept experience completed only after graduation. Further, some states may require provisional licensure of fourth-year Au.D. students in order for the experience to meet requirements, while other states do not. Again, provisional licensure is the key to the ability to bill for student services. Lack of knowledge of state provisional licensure requirements can result in students not meeting requirements for licensure or fraudulent billing of third-party payors. Without knowledge of the scope of practice as allowed by the state, students may be asked to perform services that they are not legally permitted to perform. State scope of practice, which varies from state to state, takes precedence over the scope of practice as defined by professional associations. Understanding which services students are permitted to conduct and bill for is essential to legal practice.

There are also medical-legal issues to consider. Students need to carry their own malpractice insurance, but will that absolve the preceptor of liability? That is not likely. The preceptor is responsible for assigning a task and providing supervision. In a malpractice case, the supervisor most likely will be named as a codefendent, even when appropriate supervision was provided. It is essential that preceptors interact with students on a regular basis and maintain their own malpractice insurance or ensure that they are covered under the facility's policy.

STUDENTS AND JUNIOR STAFF LEARN ETHICS BY EXAMPLE

Students' and less experienced professionals' future professional behavior will be shaped by the models of professionalism they experience clinically. The preceptor's business practices, commitment to patients, and professional interactions are likely to be emulated by the student.

Open discussion of business practices is educational. Preceptors should, through their examples and discussions, demonstrate the core ethical business values:

- You cannot help people if you do not stay in business. The practice must operate in accordance with legal standards, and the practice must be profitable.
- You cannot stay in business if you do not help people. You must be committed to patient welfare. Professionalism involves putting the patient's interest ahead of personal interests.

Students and staff need to understand that decisions about vendors are made based on the quality and cost-effectiveness of the product and the service. Ethical business people do not have conflicts of interest. They are not influenced by where the salesman takes them to lunch, and they do not accept kickbacks. Audiologists and students can gracefully accept gifts of nominal value that help remind the audiologist and student of the products and its features. Items of nominal value that enhance patient care are particularly appropriate. However, students and inexperienced audiologists may place higher value on these items due to their novelty. It may be helpful to remind them that gifts should not be accepted if one feels that it compels him or her to reciprocate the favor by ordering that vendor's product. When the student notes an increase in the number of products prescribed after a vendor visit, she or he may conclude that it is expected in reciprocity for kindnesses extended. Preceptors may wish to offer comments such as, "The sales representative's visit reminded me that this feature can benefit my patients."

Remember not only that the *Code of Ethics* requires personal compliance but that you will hold others to this standard. If either the student or preceptor is aware of unethical behavior on the part of an Academy member, he or she is obliged to report it to the Academy.

NOTE

1. The term "preceptor" will be used to refer to the audiologist supervising students; this term was recommended by the Consensus Conference on Au.D. Education. "Preceptor" connotes a teacher rather than one whose job is to supervise the autonomous actions of others.

REFERENCES

American Academy of Audiology. (2006) Position statement: audiologist's assistant. *Audiology Today* 18(2):25–26.

American Medical Association. Council on Ethical and Judicial Affairs. (2004a) Medical-student involvement in patient care [Opinion 8.087]. In: *Code of Medical Ethics: Current Opinions with Annotations, 2004-2005 Edition*. AMA Press, 224.

American Medical Association. Council on Ethical and Judicial Affairs. (2004b) Sexual harassment and exploitation between medical supervisors and trainees [Opinion 3.08]. In: *Code of Medical Ethics: Current Opinions with Annotations, 2004–2005 Edition*. AMA Press, 113.

Beauchamp T, Childress J. (1994) *Principles of Biomedical Ethics*. 4th ed. New York: Oxford University Press.

Berggren I, Severinsson E. (2003) Nurse supervisors' actions in relation to their decision-making style and ethical approach to clinical supervision. *J Adv Nurs* 41(6):615–622.

Bernard JM, Goodyear RK. (1992) *Fundamentals of Clinical Supervision*. Boston: Allyn and Bacon.

British Psychological Society. (2003) *A Briefing Paper on Sexual Harassment at Work and the Ethics of Dual Relationships*. http://www.bps.org.uk/the-society/ethics-rules-charter-code-of-conduct/code-of-conduct/a-briefing-paper-on-sexual-harassment-at-work-and-the-ethics-of-dual-relationships.cfm.

Hyrkas K, Paunonen-Ilmonen M. (2001) The effects of clinical supervision on the quality of care: examining the results of team supervision. *J Adv Nurs* 33: 492–502.

Rassi J. (1987) The uniqueness of audiology supervision. In: Crago MB, Pickering M, eds. *Supervision in Human Communication Disorders*. Boston: College Hill, 31–54.

Yager J. (N.d.) Workplace friendships or office romance. SelfGrowth.com. http://www.selfgrowth.com/articles/yager.html.

Chapter 9

Ethical Issues in Academia
Teri Hamill, Ph.D.

There are many ethical considerations in academia; however, educators may not have been exposed to all relevant areas during their training. This may be particularly true for those with professional doctorates in audiology, whose training did not include mentored teaching and research. This is not to imply that all Ph.D. students have been exposed to a diversity of ethics topics in their doctoral studies. Both Au.D. and Ph.D. academics will encounter dilemmas on the job. This chapter discusses some of the common ethical considerations.

THE PROFESSOR'S RESEARCH RESPONSIBILITIES

Research efforts help universities gain prestige, and grant money helps to fund students and purchase equipment. Scholarly research and peer-reviewed publication is an important aspect in academia; it is important to both the institution and to the individual faculty member. Research productivity is also the most important criterion for tenure at research institutions (Lucks Mendel et al, 2004).

Appendix 2 contains information on research ethics that will be of interest to the reader. However, these guidelines do not address scientific misconduct, which occurs when a researcher actively deceives others (Goodstein, 2002). The most blatant form of scientific misconduct would be to publish data known to be incorrect or fabricated, which, Goodstein (2002) reports, is relatively rare but does occur. It is reported that career pressures or the need for timely completion of studies by students typically influences the researcher to publish work that is not complete. Those who violate research ethics typically believe the results would be correct had the experiment been run to its conclusion. Fields where there is greater difficulty in replicating results tend to have greater potential for abuse.

Credit for authorship is another area of potential abuse. When conducting research with students (either as a research mentor or supervisor), one should clearly indicate which ideas are those of the student and which are the professor's.

Most of the time, research is a joint student-professor undertaking. The professor may develop the initial research proposal; the student may then add ideas. When presenting the data (either in written or oral form), it is necessary to make clear the role of both the professor and the student—and to acknowledge particular contributions of the student. In the experience of Raymond Carhart, Northwestern University, if the idea were his and he were to tell the student what to do, then he would be first author, and possibly the sole author; if the idea were his but the student were to do most of the work, then he might still be first author, but the student would definitely be included; if the student were to generate the idea but need a great deal of help, then the student would be first author and he (Carhart) would be second author; if the student were to generate the idea and do most of the research and writing independently, then he or she would be the sole author (L.A. Wilber, pers. comm.). The principle here is to give fair credit to all involved in the research study.

The American Psychological Association (2001) standard is for authorship to be granted to those who have made "substantial scientific contributions" to the study. Discussions between principal participants early in the project should clearly define what is meant by a substantial scientific contribution. A student may assume that data collection is a substantive contribution, whereas if that task could be completed by a technician and has no professional component, the effort may warrant recognition in the publication rather than authorship, as would be typical for those who perform clerical tasks. As is discussed in the *Guidelines for Ethical Practice in Research for Audiologists* (Appendix 2), early and in-depth discussion of authorship is needed.

If a student assists in data collection or analysis, it is important to consider whether the involvement benefits the student. If the student is being paid, it can be appropriate to have the student complete work that is not directly related to his or her needs. If the student is not receiving direct funding from the research, one must consider how much of the effort is directed toward meeting the professor's professional goals (e.g., for tenure or promotion) and how much the professor is truly helping the student learn about the research process.

Sometimes, academic supervisors place such high value on research that there is pressure to expend energies in that pursuit at the expense of other equally important activities (McElroy and Rassi, 1992), such as student teaching. Audiology is a rapidly changing health-care profession, and faculty members frequently teach a number of different courses each year. They have an ethical responsibility to provide students current information in each course, which can be time-consuming because of the large number of courses that must be taught.

Universities differ in their teaching and research expectations, and in their allowance for course preparation time. Before accepting an employment offer, it is prudent to ask the department chair, college dean, and other faculty members about specific expectations and release time policies. As a professor, teaching classes in the research interest area is an excellent way to ensure that information taught is current.

COMMUNICATING SCHOLARLY INFORMATION

Good teaching and good clinical supervision are not easy. The task is made even more challenging in that many academics have not received training in how to teach or supervise (McElroy and Rassi, 1992). Both require excellent communication skills, which involves introducing new concepts as simply as possible, while providing the greatest possible depth and breadth of education (American Association of University Professors [AAUP], 1987). Students enroll in academic programs for a limited time; the professor's responsibility is to facilitate their learning and develop their critical thinking skills during that time frame. This is a tremendous responsibility; professors and faculty are entrusted with the education of the next generation of audiologists. The quality of the student's academic preparation impacts the health care received by the patients of the future audiologist.

A faculty member may be asked to teach courses or provide clinical supervision in an area in which he or she is inadequately prepared. If this occurs, it is important for the faculty member to talk with the department chair to make sure that he or she understands the faculty member's limitations. However, it is not appropriate to refuse to teach a course for which one has been trained simply because the material is not interesting. Ideally, all universities would have enough faculty so that each faculty member would only be asked to teach those courses in which they are expert. Although ideal, this is unlikely to happen. Again, it is preferable to have reached agreement on teaching and supervision loads before accepting a faculty position. However, after the contract has been signed, one must recognize that sometimes the needs of the department change, affecting the professor's work assignments.

If accepting research or administrative responsibilities that permit release from teaching responsibilities, the professor and department chair have an ethical responsibility to ensure that the person teaching the course is adequately prepared. Graduate teaching assistants who are new to teaching and newly hired personnel with limited or no teaching experience will require mentoring. While providing syllabi and teaching materials may be helpful and appreciated, the new instructor may lack skills in communicating the information. Direct observation and mentoring are necessary and appropriate.

Different clinical and teaching faculty may have varied clinical philosophies and approaches. Beginning students often express frustration that no two instructors agree on everything and no two preceptors use exactly the same procedures. When students understand the rationale behind differences in procedures, they are more enthusiastic about experimenting with them. If there appears to be a specific way in which other clinical faculty/staff conduct a particular test or selection procedure, it is appropriate to ask why that method is used and to discuss it as one of the appropriate approaches in class or use it as a clinical technique. If the test or procedure is not supported by the literature, that should be discussed directly with the faculty/staff person, rather than placing the student in an uncomfortable position.

CONFLICTS OF INTEREST AND STUDENT EVALUATION

The cynical Paul Trout said regarding course evaluations that "analysis of the content of and student responses to college course evaluations suggests that, in general, students are seeking entertainment, comfort, high grades, and less work and are hostile to the necessary routines and rigors of higher education. The commonly used numerical evaluation form is not only unreliable and invalid, it is an effective device for lowering academic standards" (1997, p. 24). There is evidence to refute this claim (e.g., Kulik, 2001), but anyone with teaching experience will recognize the grain of truth in Trout's statement. If one's motivation is to attain high course evaluation ratings, these sometimes can be achieved at the expense of academic rigor. Some students rate "easy 'A'" courses highly.

Grade inflation pressures have to be resisted. Employers need to be able to review a student transcript and recognize which student is good and which student is excellent. They need assurance that those who graduate are academically qualified for practice. The academic audiologist's responsibility is to challenge their students and to reward excellence.

Some clinicians perceive academic faculty as having an inherent conflict of interest in grading students. Without a sufficient number of students, the academic program will not be supported. A disreputable university might accept underqualified students and retain them so the faculty has employment. The presumption that this is common is as ludicrous as the idea that practitioners will dispense hearing aids that do not benefit patients in order to stay employed. As long as beneficence is the underlying motive, no conflict of interest exists (Resnick, 1993a). If the faculty's motive is to educate students, there is no reason they should not be remunerated for the effort, just as being paid to provide clinical services is entirely ethical. Of course it is unethical for admissions committees to accept students who are unlikely to succeed. It is not in the marginal student's interest to allow him or her to languish in the program only to be dismissed in the later years of study.

Professors need to serve as gatekeepers. Not all students are excellent; not all students accepted into a program will attain sufficient proficiency to graduate. It is emotionally difficult to inform a student that he or she has not passed a course. It is painful to have to advise a student that his or her clinical skills do not appear to be advancing adequately. These tasks, however difficult, are a faculty member's responsibility.

It is also important to consider the grade recommendations of off-campus preceptors adequately and appropriately. A student who appears to do very well (or very poorly) on campus may receive the opposite evaluation from off-campus preceptors. It is important to talk with the off-campus preceptors to understand what their expectations were and how the student did or did not reach them. Use of the model suggested by Rassi (1987; Rassi and McElroy, 1992), in which clear expectations are developed for students by quarter/semester, may facilitate understanding between the faculty and off-campus preceptors. If the on- and off-campus preceptors (and the student) are in agreement about the expectations, there are likely to be few if any disagreements about the performance evaluation.

It is also important to know the specific types of cases that were seen by each student at his or her off-campus placement, which can be determined by direct observation, or communication via telephone or e-mail. Sometimes a placement will not provide an adequate number of cases to evaluate certain performance (e.g., contralateral masking for patients with conductive hearing loss). In that case, evaluation differences may be understood—but they still need to be reconciled. If the faculty does not adequately consider the grade recommendations of these off-campus preceptors, the student will not receive optimal feedback, and eventually, perhaps, the preceptor will be less likely to accept student placements because their input on student performance was not adequately considered.

When recommending a student for an external placement or for employment, it is important to honestly describe a student's abilities and limitations. If a letter of recommendation does not support the student for that placement, the faculty member should inform the student. Providing a less than complete and honest evaluation of that student's strengths and weaknesses can damage the reputation of the professor and the institution and, ultimately, is not helpful to the student. Particularly in this litigious environment, it is important to respect the student's right to privacy. Recommendations should not be provided without the student's consent, ideally in writing. The authorization and a copy of the letter of recommendation may best be stored in the student's confidential departmental file.

TEACHING ETHICS AND UPHOLDING ACADEMIC INTEGRITY

Ideally, ethics would be infused throughout the audiology curriculum. There are opportunities to discuss ethical issues in classes on research as well as in diagnostic and treatment courses. Courses could include a module that examines how the national professional organizations and state regulations address ethical issues.

Academic integrity has to be taught, as students generally do not understand what is and is not acceptable. The essay in the text box on the following page, "Advice to Students on Avoiding Plagiarism," may be a useful reference for educating students about plagiarism and appropriate referencing. Surprisingly, many students truly do not know what constitutes plagiarism. In this electronic age, high-school students may have used the Internet for research, and it may have been considered acceptable "research" for students to "cut and paste" information into their submissions, without putting the material in their own

ADVICE TO STUDENTS ON AVOIDING PLAGIARISM
Laura Ann Wilber, Ph.D.

Be careful to avoid any suspicion of plagiarism. According to *Webster's*,[1] to "plagiarize" is "to steal and pass off (the ideas or words of another) as one's own: use (another's production) without crediting the source." Northwestern University's description of dishonesty in academic work includes the following statement: "plagiarism: submitting material that in part or whole is not entirely one's own work without attributing those same portions to their correct source" (Northwestern University, 1992). To avoid the appearance of plagiarism, it is important to document (especially in term papers) every statement that cannot be considered to be *general knowledge*. I realize that this can get in the way of a smooth flow of ideas, and so in journal articles sometimes authors wait until the end of a long section before making such references. In term papers, it is usually better (unless your professor tells you otherwise) to over-reference rather than under-reference. I know of *no* case when listing a group of references only at the end of a paper would be considered adequate documentation.

If you use the exact wording found in your source, you must put it in quotation marks and indicate the page number as well as the specific source:

> For example: "the values of the scores obtained on speech intelligibility tests are influenced by the proficiency and training of the talker and listening crew, as well as the difficulty of the speech material being used. Therefore, one cannot expect that a given communication system will provide identical test scores when tested in different laboratories" (Kryter 1985, p. 92).

If you paraphrase, you need not use the page number, but you must cite the specific source:

> Since the particular talker/listener combination, as well as the specific speech material, will influence test results, one may obtain different scores for a unique communication system from one time and place to another (Kryter, 1985).

If several persons said the same thing, you may list more than one source after a statement:

> Many authors have mentioned the importance of the talker/material combination when considering speech recognition scores (Lehiste and Peterson, 1965; Kryter, 1985; Dirks, 1986; Rintelmann, 1990).

NOTE

1. *Merriam-Webster's Collegiate Dictionary*, 11th ed., s.v. "Plagiarize."

REFERENCE

Northwestern University. (1992) *Principles Regarding Academy Integrity.* http://www.northwestern.edu/uacc/uniprin.html.

words. Appropriate referencing of information, regardless of its source, and the importance of using one's own wording need to be taught. Rennie and Rudland (2003) reported that 77 percent of medical students saw nothing wrong with copying directly from texts or articles, as long as the source was cited, and 18 percent believed it was acceptable to do so without a citation. Approximately 15 percent admitted to plagiarizing or contemplating plagiarism. Clearly, students need instruction on avoiding plagiarism.

When they are told they should not include extensive direct quotes in their papers, students may think an acceptable alternative is to replace a few words with synonyms, adopting the original sentence structure and much of its verbiage. One method of teaching what is, and is not, acceptable is by having students read short original article segments and various synopses, and identify which summaries are and are not acceptable. It may be prudent to test on this concept to ensure that it is understood before students write their first paper. In spite of these efforts, there will be students who include plagiarized material in their first literature review paper. This is not a problem unique to audiology; it has also been problematic across disciplines.

Assigning specific paper topics or report requirements may lessen the chance that the student can purchase a paper online; however, it will not stop the student from plagiarizing from their reference sources. When assigning literature review papers, monitoring student progress throughout the semester will help to discourage the procrastination that can lead to last-minute plagiarism. For example, the professor may wish to review the outline and rough draft of the student's literature review. It is also helpful to require students to submit the articles used in writing the papers (complete with original highlighting). This way, when the paper has uneven writing—segments of writing typical of the beginning student, interspersed with brilliant phrasing—the professor can readily compare the submission to the referenced article's text. Additionally, if the professor retains a copy of the submitted papers, he or she is able to make comparisons to subsequent student submissions.

Software programs are available that will compare the electronic student submission to other reference texts. Some of these services require that the professor submit electronic copies of the student papers to expand the available data bank. This raises ethical and legal questions (Howard, 2003). The student is the owner of his or her own copyright, having authored the material. He or she should have the ability to determine the use of his or her intellectual property. While the professor may trust the site, it is possible that the material submitted could be used inappropriately.

Cheating on tests appears to be widespread. Kvam (1996) reported that 18 percent of college students cheated on the statistics exam administered during the study. It is unwise to assume that students in health-care professions will refrain from temptation. Five to ten percent of medical students cheat, and one study reported that 5.5 percent of optometry students admitted to cheating during their professional studies, with 14 percent cheating sometime during their college career (Werner et al, 2000). Vigilance by the professor appears to be a necessary precaution.

Kerkvliet and Sigmund (1999) evaluated the factors that reduce the risk of cheating. While some believe avoiding multiple-choice test questions and increasing the physical spacing between students is helpful, their research did not support those assumptions. They report cheating to be more common when graduate teaching assistants were responsible for a class: Students were 32 percent less likely to cheat when a faculty member taught that section of the course. Use of multiple versions of a test (e.g., distributing two test versions with questions in different order) reduced cheating, as did verbal warnings given prior to the test and having multiple test proctors.

Students may not consider it cheating to review the graded exams of more senior students, particularly if the professor does not explicitly prohibit them from doing so. Even if the professor creates new questions each semester, if some students have access to old exams and others do not, those students who do are unfairly advantaged. Collecting exams after the students have reviewed them eliminates this problem; however, the disadvantage to this approach is that students do not have their graded tests to use in study for final exams, comprehensive exams, or the exam administered by credentialing bodies. An alternative approach is to provide last year's exams to all students. Students should be informed that the exam focus can change and that any exam is a sampling of their knowledge; that is, a concept not tested last year could appear on this year's exam, and concepts tested last year may not be queried.

ACCEPTING SERVICE RESPONSIBILITIES

While the board of directors, provosts, president, and university administration have management responsibilities, they typically share control over the academic integrity of the university with the faculty. Committees that oversee new programs and changes in curriculum, the institutional review board, the faculty senate, and tenure and promotion committees are among those that figure prominently in assuring university quality. Universities retain their academic integrity and faculties retain their academic freedom because of faculty participation in these governance functions (AAUP, 1987). Faculty may find mentors or research collaborators among the committee members. Learning the values and culture of the university is also a likely outcome of committee participation. This can help junior faculty in understanding the university's mores and requirements for tenure, which might influence them in deciding whether this university is the right professional home.

While committee participation has advantages to junior faculty, limited participation is advised in the early years. Universities recognize that tremendous effort is required to teach new courses and establish a research program. Expectations for committee involvement are greater for senior faculties, who have a responsibility to accept a greater role in governance and committee work (Lucks Mendel et al, 2004).

Service to professional organizations is also an obligation; membership-driven organizations such as the American Academy of Audiology (Academy) rely on volunteers. Universities traditionally expect professional service of senior faculty members and, as such, may make some allowance in workloads. The flexibility in the academic audiologist's schedule provides opportunities to serve on Academy committees that those in other practice settings may not enjoy. The networking opportunities this service provides are a reward, as is the satisfaction of knowing that you help guide your profession.

THE IMPACT OF FACULTY DEPARTURE ON STUDENTS

Faculty decisions to leave a university dramatically impact students, particularly those involved in collaborative research and those whose dissertations or theses the professor chairs. When possible, faculty should plan their departures well in advance and inform colleagues and students (AAUP, 1987). When feasible, faculty should offer to continue advising students and serving on research evaluation committees after leaving the university. This can be very helpful to the student and might prevent the student from having to redo a substantial portion of the dissertation research (L.A. Wilber, pers. comm., 2004).

Realistically, the process of hiring replacement faculty requires a six-month to one-year effort. In recent years, some searches have extended beyond a year due to Ph.D. personnel shortages, particularly in high-demand specialties. The position must be advertised and applicants interviewed, and those applicants will wish to give their current employers adequate notice of their intentions. Leaving an academic position with little notice, particularly in the middle of a semester, is unprofessional and likely to impact the professor's reputation negatively.

STUDENT/PROFESSOR RELATIONSHIPS

The concepts discussed in Chapter 8 concerning preceptor/student relationships hold true for professors as well. It is important for faculty to retain objectivity and to ensure that students are not placed in uncomfortable situations. It is also important to recognize that, sometimes, cultural differences may exist between the professor and a student that change the student's expectations of appropriate interaction.

USE ACADEMIC AFFILIATIONS PRUDENTLY

The Academy *Code of Ethics* (*COE*; see pp. xv–xxi of this book) Rule 8b prescribes that "individuals shall not engage in dishonesty or illegal conduct that adversely reflects on the profession." If the public recognizes a professional as an audiologist, the professional's personal conduct in public reflects on the profession (Resnick, 1993b). This concept holds equally true in regard to the university. The faculty member's friends and neighbors likely know him or her both as an audiologist and as a professor. Personal conduct reflects, positively or negatively, on the university.

Traditionally, professors publicly use their academic affiliation only in professional contexts (AAUP, 1987). For example, an audiologist would not sign a letter to the editor analyzing a current news event with "Assistant Professor, State University," although a political science faculty member might. If interviewed on a topic related to audiology, for example, about the efficacy of canalith repositioning maneuvers, the professor should ask the reporter to note his or her university affiliation. One should be cautious, though, not to appear to speak for the university. The university may request that faculty contact the public affairs office before speaking with the press.

APPROPRIATE USE OF EVALUATION COPIES OF TEXTBOOKS

Upon request, textbook publishers will provide teaching faculty with evaluation or "desk" copies of texts so that professors can determine whether that text is appropriate for adoption. This is widespread practice across disciplines. The publisher's intent is to encourage faculty to explore alternative texts in the hopes that a new offering may prove beneficial. Hamill et al (2001) asked different groups for their perception of what is and is not ethical, and included questions about textbooks. While students were not necessarily happy to learn that professors get free books, 38 of the 40 students felt the practice was acceptable.

The acceptance of free desk copies raises potential ethics concerns. Typically, publishers in audiology provide desk copies without purchase commitment. Some publishers stipulate that the text is only free if an order for the text is placed. This could create a situation where the instructor, who wishes to retain the free text, decides to adopt it for a semester, even if it is not ideal for the course. Unquestionably, that would be unethical. In order for the professor to avoid the appearance of conflict of interest, evaluation copies should not be accepted if a "string" is attached, as per the Academy *COE*.

Text publishers want their books evaluated for potential adoption. They do not, however, want to stock professors' professional libraries for free. In preparing material for this article, the author asked major publishers in audiology their opinions on desk copies. With only a few responses, the results cannot be generalized, but trends were evident. The less likely an evaluation copy will be an adopted course text, the more unethical it is of the professor to request it. Do publishers want professors to request a desk copy if there is a 50 percent chance of adoption? What if the text was optional? What if there is only a slight chance it will be selected as an optional text? There is no complete agreement across publishers, but by the time the scenario involved a 25 percent chance that the text would be adopted as an optional course resource, the respondents did not approve. It is appropriate to let the publisher know how the desk copy will be utilized. The publisher may be willing to provide a courtesy copy, even if it is not probable that the text will be adopted.

How do you dispose of an unwanted desk copy? If upon review, the text is not appropriate, should it be returned? Surprisingly, that is not requested. One publisher's representative explained that postage and restocking/handling expenses would be greater than the cost of printing the book. However, it is not their intent for the free text to prevent another sale. One sales representative, who asked to remain anonymous, offered the following opinion on how to dispose of texts that a professor no longer cares to retain.

> NEVER, NEVER, NEVER sell a book to the used book buyer who haunts the halls. This is the height of unprofessional behavior. When professors sell books given as samples for course consideration, they are costing the publisher money, as the opportunity to sell a new book may be obviated. The publisher cannot recover costs, the author will be deprived of royalties, and the real cost of books to the student is increased because someone has to pay for the cost of samples. . . . Professors who sell books to used book merchants are hurting their profession, their colleagues, and their students. . . . If you don't want a book, give it to a library in a third world country.

CONFLICT OF INTEREST IN REQUIRING YOUR OWN TEXT

University conflict of interest guidelines will set criteria for when it is permissible for faculty to profit from sales to students. In the Hamill et al (2001) study mentioned above, 31 of 40 students felt it was unacceptable for professors to require a text from which the professor profited. One potential method of reducing the inherent conflict of interest is to calculate the amount of royalty received from the publisher for each text, and give this amount to each student or make a donation in the amount to a scholarship fund or the university library (AAUP, 2004).

COPYRIGHT REGULATIONS

Generally, any original arrangement of words can be copyrighted. An exception to this is blank forms, such as case history forms (Silverman, 1999). Thus, articles and books are copyrighted, and fair-use provisions apply. Professors and students are allowed to make copies of copyrighted material, so long as the copying does not effectively harm the owner of the copyright. The general interpretation has been that limited copying of articles or segments of articles for class is permitted. Students can, of course, make copies of journal articles for their own use. However, collecting sets of readings and copying them for students for use in lieu of a textbook cannot be done without permission from the copyright holders.

In general, if a teacher is acting "spontaneously," preparing materials so close to the class time that copyright permission cannot be secured, the professor would be allowed to copy a figure from an article, and perhaps one entire article from a journal, with proper notation indicating that the material is copyrighted. In subsequent years teaching the class, it is assumed that copyright permission will be obtained (University of Texas, 2001). Professors are encouraged to understand and follow their university's interpretation of the copyright rules. Materials from the Internet are also copyrighted. The same general principles apply (Montecino, 1996). Impromptu use is permitted with citation; routine use requires permission.

RELATIONSHIPS WITH MANUFACTURERS

Academic audiologists may request the help of manufacturers in the education of their students. The support may be through donation of equipment or via student training. There are ethical considerations in both cases.

Universities are nonprofit institutions, and manufacturers may elect to make donations, which may have tax advantages as well as marketing advantages. While it is generous of manufacturers to donate to universities, when the donations are other than unrestricted grants, there are potential concerns. Did all companies have equal opportunity to donate equipment and thus have the chance to influence impressionable students? Does receipt of equipment create a social or contractual obligation to dispense that manufacturer's product, or recommend that equipment to students? If so, the situation is a conflict of interest and not permitted given the Academy *COE*.

Donation acceptance that does not require any form of purchase commitment could still be inappropriate. For example, if the clinic conducts hearing aid evaluations where patients listen to competing hearing aids before deciding on the one to recommend, then dispensing only the brands of hearing aid whose demonstration models were provided at no cost constitutes a conflict of interest. The patient's welfare is given secondary consideration to the economic advantage, for the clinic, of not having to purchase the demonstration aids.

The Academy's *Ethical Practice Guidelines on Financial Incentives from Hearing Instrument Manufacturers* (Appendix 1) also applies to student members of the Academy. Students who accept manufacturer-sponsored training invitations should follow these guidelines. While it is preferable that travel expenses be paid by the students, if the trip is solely educational and the training cannot be accomplished at the university by a company representative, then it is permissible for the manufacturer to pay for the student travel. The conflict of interest restrictions apply, however. The accommodations must be modest, and the student should not accept manufacturer-sponsored entertainment. It would be appropriate for faculty to review these guidelines with students when training opportunities arise.

Faculty members also need to impress upon the students that manufacturer-sponsored training is credible and worthwhile if it expands and enhances the capabilities of the student in regard to the use of the commercial product they represent. It is good business for the manufacturer to encourage correct product applications and usage in order for the product to be received favorably by both the audiologist and the patient for whom it is intended. As in all things, however, the best interests of the patient should be held paramount, and any sense of obligation the student feels based on travel provided by a manufacturer should be tempered by this premise. Impressionable young professionals should not develop a sense of entitlement based on manufacturer largess, nor should they be unduly influenced by the exposure to one manufacturer's products.

Faculty members are advised to ensure that students understand their professional obligation to make the most of the learning experience by fully participating in the educational sessions, and they should be required to report what they have learned to the faculty, clinical supervisors, and other students. Unprofessional student behavior outside of the university reflects poorly on the faculty. Faculty expectations should be clear to students attending manufacturer-sponsored training.

In contrast, the American Medical Association (AMA) imposes more stringent restrictions on medical students and residents. The AMA permits medical companies to provide grants to the medical school. The faculty selects the recipients and disperses the money to offset the training expenses. Sponsorships to attend regional and national conventions are permitted, but sponsorship of student-oriented training sessions or payment of travel to industry-sponsored seminars is disallowed (American Medical Association, Council on Ethical and Judicial Affairs, 2004).

STUDENT USE OF THE TERM "Au.D. CANDIDATE"

While the term "Ph.D. candidate" has traditionally been used by those who are "all but dissertation," students in varying levels of their Au.D. programs have used the term "Au.D. candidate," which is at best misleading. Osborne (2004) points out that other doctoral-level health-care professions refer to students as "students," and urges the adoption of the more medical model. He considers this " 'wanna be' behavior" "inappropriate and embarrassing" (2004, p. 14). In January 2005, the Academy's Board of Directors accepted the following ethical advisory statement:

Student members have used the term "Au.D. candidate," which the Ethical Practice Board and Board of Directors feel is inappropriate. Use of the term "Au.D. candidate" is not consistent with first professional degrees, regardless of the student's academic standing, and use of the term is not consistent with the recommendations of the Consensus Conference on Au.D. Education. Attempts to restrict the use to those who have completed the majority of the degree requirements would likely result in disparity of the qualifications among those allowed by their university to use the term. Therefore, there should be no public use of the term "Au.D. candidate" while a person is a student.

COMPETITION WITH COMMUNITY AUDIOLOGISTS

Some in the private sector believe that university clinics utilize taxpayer support to an unfair advantage, because the university clinic expenses are offset by student tuition revenue and other state funds. Conversely, faculty may believe that student tuition and the university's provision of capital equipment serve to offset the high cost of student training and seldom subsidize the price of hearing aids for patients seen in the university clinic. Most academic clinics must be self-supporting, and often the revenue a clinic generates contributes to the overall departmental budget. The reality today is that most public university budgets have undergone continual cuts, so that university programs are less able to rely on state and federal funding. A private practice has an economic advantage in that the professional staff functions efficiently and patient care is provided more expeditiously. In the university clinic, direct supervision of beginning-level students, who require considerably more time with each patient, is an expensive proposition.

It is wise for the staff of university clinics to fully consider the costs of providing services and dispensing hearing instruments in order to set fair prices. This maximizes the likelihood that community audiologists will agree to serve as external site preceptors. Community audiologists will be unwilling to act as preceptors if students are not properly trained before leaving on-site training. It is difficult for students to gain proficiency within an active, full-service, nonuniversity clinic or practice if said students have not received adequate clinical experience during rotations within the university clinic. Therefore, community audiologists generally support state-of-the-art university training facilities where students gain exposure and preparation in the full scope of practice, so long as the university clinic does not have fees that are substantially less than those in the community, and as long as the university clinic freely accepts their share of indigent patients.

While advocating that university clinics price competitively, it is wise to be mindful of price-fixing prohibitions. Government regulations prohibit collusion in setting prices; therefore, clinical faculty cannot directly ask the audiologists in the community about their pricing structure. National data can help determine typical costs for procedures and products, and calculation of the clinic's costs of service provision, including overhead, can also be used in establishing fees and prices.

ETHICAL FINANCIAL DEALING WITH THE UNIVERSITY

Some universities recognize that the salaries they pay are not competitive with the private sector and permit "faculty clinics," where the faculty members earn additional income working in a university-supported practice. Most universities are not so generous. While it might be tempting to use university facilities after hours for personal gain, the university's approval must be obtained.

University (and other) clinics have regulations on how money is spent. Especially in hard economic times, continuing education, travel budgets, and capital equipment lines are limited. In some cases, clinic administrators have been able to negotiate use of clinic revenues for these types of expenses. The Ethical Practice Board (EPB) recently heard from an administrator who was not so fortunate. This audiologist used a buying group that agreed to invoice the university at the single unit rate for hearing instruments. The buying group set aside a certain amount per instrument dispensed and deposited it in an account that could be used for expenses that the institution restricted. The EPB advised the member to immediately cease and desist. While the EPB assumed the audiologist considered the benefits of enhanced equipment and well-educated staff the greater good, this was an obvious violation of the institution's policy. If discovered, it could result in dismissal and in criminal action. Other staff members might have concerns about their supervisor's use of these funds. If the institution no longer has oversight of the expenditures and the administrator was willing to bend rules, inappropriate personal use of funds could easily occur.

LEADING BY EXAMPLE

Audiologists typically have held academic faculty in high regard. The EPB asks faculty to help lead the profession and continue to earn its well-placed respect by remaining at the forefront of personal and professional ethical practice. We hope that professors will endeavor to instill ethical values in those who seek to join the profession.

REFERENCES

American Academy of Audiology. (2005) Ethical Practice Board advisory: use of the term "AuD candidate" deemed inappropriate. *Audiol Today* 17(2):45.

American Association of University Professors (AAUP). (1987) *Statement on Professional Ethics.* http://www.aaup.org/statements/Redbook/Rbethics.htm.

American Association of University Professors (AAUP). (2004) *On Professors Assigning Their Own Texts to Students.* http://www.aaup.org/statements/REPORTS/AssignOwnText.htm.

American Medical Association. Council on Ethical and Judicial Affairs. (2004) Gifts to physicians from industry and clarification [Opinion 8.061]. In: *Code of Medical Ethics: Current Opinions with Annotations, 2004–2005 Edition.* AMA Press, 203–214.

American Psychological Association. (2001) Ethical standards for the reporting and publishing of scientific information. In: *Publication Manual of the American Psychological Association.* Washington, DC: American Psychological Association, 387–396.

Goodstein D. (2002) Scientific misconduct. *Academe* 88(1). http://www.aaup.org/publications/Academe/2002/02JF/02jfgoo.htm.

Hamill T, Doyle L, Freeman B. (2001) Ethics / professionalism: avoid being voted off the island. Instructional course at the annual meeting of the American Academy of Audiology, San Diego.

Howard RM. (2003) The search for a cure: understanding the "plagiarism epidemic." McGraw Hill. http://www.mhhe.com/socscience/english/tc/howard/HowardModule03.htm.

Kerkvliet J, Sigmund CL. (1999) Can we control cheating in the classroom? *J Econ Educ* 30(4):331–343.

Kulik J. (2001) Student ratings: validity, utility and controversy. *New Dir Inst Res* 109(Spring):9–25.

Kvam PH. (1996) Using exam scores to estimate the prevalence of classroom cheating. *Am Stat* 50(3):238–243.

Lucks Mendel L, Mendel MI, Battle DE. (2004) Climbing the academic ladder. *ASHA Leader* 9(14):1, 6–7, 23.

McElroy MD, Rassi JA. (1992) Learning teaching, improving teaching. In: *The Education of Audiologists and Speech-Language Pathologists*. Timonium, MD: York Press, 3–30.

Montecino V. (1996) Copyright and the internet. http://mason.gmu.edu/~montecin/copyright-internet.htm

Osborne GS. (2004) State of audiology: feature. *ADA Feedback* 15(2):13–15.

Rassi JA. (1987) The uniqueness of audiology supervision. In: Crago MB, Pickering M, eds. *Supervision in Human Communication Disorders: Perspectives on a Process*. Boston: Little, Brown, 31–53.

Rassi JA, McElroy MD. (1992) Clinical teaching: delineating competencies and planning strategies. In: Rassi JA, McElroy MD, eds. *The Education of Audiologists and Speech-Language Pathologists*. Timonium, MD: York Press, 301–335.

Rennie SC, Rudland JR. (2003) Differences in medical students' attitudes to academic misconduct and reported behavior across the years—a questionnaire study. *J Med Ethics* 29:97–102.

Resnick DM. (1993a) The code of ethics. In: *Professional Ethics for Audiologists and Speech-Language Pathologists*. San Diego: Singular Publishing, 17–38.

Resnick DM. (1993b) Jurisdiction, diversity and some other ethical concerns. In: *Professional Ethics for Audiologists and Speech-Language Pathologists*. San Diego: Singular Publishing, 55–70.

Silverman FH. (1999) Copyright considerations for clinicians. *Professional Issues in Speech Language Pathology and Audiology*. Boston: Allyn and Bacon, 177–185.

Trout P. (1997) What the numbers mean: providing a context for numerical student evaluations of courses. *Change* 29(5):24–30.

University of Texas. (2001) Guidelines for classroom copying of books and periodicals. http://www.utsystem.edu/ogc/intellectualproperty/clasguid.htm.

Werner DL, Hejberger MH, Feldman J, Johnston E. (2000) The prevalence of unethical student behavior in optometry schools. Abstract. *Optom Educ* 25(3):82–87.

Chapter 10

Procedures of the Ethical Practice Board: Frequently Asked Questions
Jane M. Kukula, Au.D.
Teri Hamill, Ph.D.

Q: I have an ethics question, not a complaint. Does the Ethical Practice Board provide any help?

A: Yes. When a member is faced with an ethical dilemma, the Ethical Practice Board (EPB) may be able to provide assistance. This book and other EPB articles and publications contain information on many aspects of ethical practice in audiology. While the main intent of these materials is to further educate audiologists in the area of ethics, they can also be used for reference when analyzing ethical questions. The American Academy of Audiology (Academy) Web site (http://www.audiology.org/) has links to many of these ethics resources. After reviewing this information, if one is still uncertain as to how to proceed, members may seek input on the issue directly from the EPB. Specific questions or issues can be e-mailed to the EPB at ethics@audiology.org or mailed to the following address:

Chair, EPB
American Academy of Audiology
11730 Plaza American Drive, Suite 300
Reston, VA 20190

Q: I have read the procedures in the Academy *Code of Ethics*, but I'm not sure that I understand the sequence.

A: The flowchart in Figure 1 may help. Not included in the flowchart is the EPB's method of communicating to the original complainant. The complainant is not informed of the EPB decision, except when the EPB decides not to pursue the case. In all other cases, the complainant is informed that the matter has been deliberated and that, due to privacy concerns, the complainant cannot be informed of the decision reached. (The *Code of Ethics [COE]* appears on pages xv–xxi of this book.)

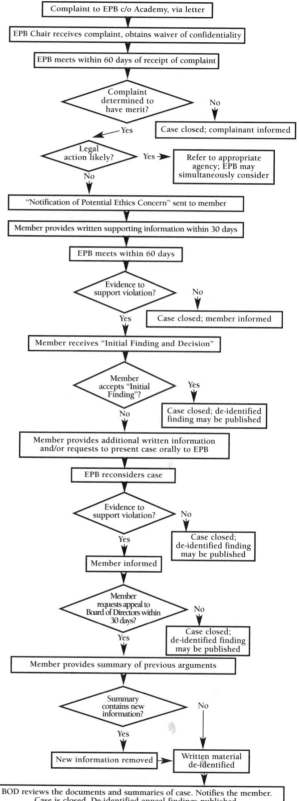

Figure 1.
Complaint sequence.

Q: I think something is an ethical violation. What should I do?

A: While it can be uncomfortable to report your concerns about another colleague, self-regulation is a professional responsibility and an expectation of those in an autonomous profession. Rule 8c of the *COE* reads: "Individuals shall inform the Ethical Practice Board when there are reasons to believe that a member of the Academy may have violated the Code of Ethics."

Q: Do I have to give my name when I report a suspected ethical violation?

A: Without knowledge of the identity of the complainant, if the information is inadequate, the EPB may not be able to obtain clarification and therefore may not be able to take action. While the EPB asks that you provide your name and contact information, your name does not have to be provided to the person suspected of having violated the *COE*. Complainants are asked to sign a waiver of confidentiality, allowing the EPB to use their name when discussing the allegations with the complainant. However, the member has the right not to sign the waiver. In this case, only the Academy's Executive Director, staff designated by the Executive Director, and the EPB will know your identity.

Q: The membership renewal form asks if I've had a state licensure violation. If I report that I have, will that affect my membership?

A: Members are required to provide accurate information. Certainly, not reporting or intentionally providing incorrect information will have a negative effect on membership. Informing the Academy of discipline by a state does not automatically mean membership will be affected. The nature of the infraction and the discipline will be reviewed by the EPB. Following EPB consideration, either the case will be closed or the member will receive a request for further information. If the EPB believes it is necessary to investigate the matter further, the member will be offered the opportunity to explain events and extenuating circumstances. Probation (where membership benefits are retained so long as the member complies with the stipulated consent agreement) and suspension and revocation of membership are the harshest penalties available to the EPB and are used for discipline for the severest ethical violations. A member who self-reports an ethical violation or licensure violation has taken a critical step in admitting to an error or lapse of judgment. In many cases, the member's report is sufficient, and no further action is taken.

Q: I just received a "Notification of Potential Ethics Concern." I'll be honest, I'm mad, and I'm scared. I don't want my name dragged through the mud.

A: The EPB maintains confidentiality of personal information. If the worse case scenario occurs and a member is found to be in violation of the *COE*, only the information regarding the member's actions and the violation would be released. Often, when no finding is reached, no information is ever published. However, the circumstances of your case may be published, even if you are not found to be in violation, if doing so would help members to understand what is, and is not, permitted within the *COE*. In either case, your name would not be disclosed during deliberations to anyone other than the Academy Executive Director, staff designated by the Executive Director, and the EPB, and your name would not appear in any published report about the case.

Q: Where do these complaints come from?

A: The EPB receives complaints from consumers, members, and the Academy staff. Members are obliged by the *COE* to report suspected violations. Additionally, the Academy asks state licensure and registration boards to provide information on members who have had action against their license.

Q: Should I involve my lawyer? Is it better for the lawyer to communicate with the EPB or for me to write directly?

A: Certainly a member can involve an attorney, but that is usually not necessary. In the initial stages of a complaint, the EPB is simply looking for information and is attempting to determine what happened and if the complaint has merit. If after reviewing the information it is determined that there may have been a violation, the member is afforded the opportunity to explain and "argue their case."

Q: Can I call someone to talk about this? I'm better at explaining my side of the story orally.

A: When responding to the "Notification of Potential Ethics Concern," you need to reply in writing. This way you are not relying on someone else to relay the information accurately, and all EPB members receive all of the information. If the written information you initially provided does not satisfy the EPB, and you are given an "Initial Finding" with which you disagree, you will have the opportunity to discuss the matter orally. You will be able to present information either at a face-to-face meeting of the EPB or in a teleconference call. If you appeal your case to the Board of Directors (BOD), the appeal must be in written format.

  If one has procedural questions, contacting the EPB Chair is appropriate. Contact with other EPB members is discouraged. Discussion of a case outside of EPB deliberations may be cause for an EPB member to recuse him- or herself.

Q: How much information do I need to provide?

A: Please provide a full, yet succinct, report. Carefully answer all points raised. It is not necessary, nor is it helpful, to include additional information, such as testimonials from patients or colleagues, or your curriculum vitae or publications, unless that information directly relates to the concern. For example, if questioned about professional competence, including reports of CEU activities is appropriate. That information would not be helpful if the concern was a violation of conflict of interest guidelines.

Q: How do you decide on the penalty that should be invoked?

A: Though discipline needs to be based on the violation, individual circumstances are considered. The EPB considers the severity of the violation, whether it was inadvertent or intentional, the member's attitude, and the level of cooperation. Also, discipline can be progressive. Whether the member has been disciplined previously or whether the violation under review is a repeat offense are questions considered by the EPB.

Q: Do decisions by the EPB have to be unanimous?

A: No, only a majority vote of a quorum of the nine board members is needed to discipline a member. The exception is the penalty of membership revocation, which requires a two-thirds majority.

Q: What are the procedures to follow when I receive the "Notification of Potential Ethics Concern"?

A: Following the receipt of a notice, one has 30 days to respond, in writing, to the concerns included in the letter. This is your initial opportunity to provide information. Send any relevant supporting documentation you may have. If the EPB is satisfied at this point, the case may be closed.

Q: If I have other problems and I really can't respond right away, will you give a deadline extension?

A: One must respond to the request within 30 days. If there are extenuating circumstances such as debilitating illness, contact the EPB chair to discuss your options as soon as possible.

Q: I responded to the "Notification of Potential Ethics Concern," and yet I was sent an "Initial Finding and Decision" that indicates that the EPB still thinks I have violated the *Code of Ethics*, and a penalty has been proposed. I don't agree with the "Initial Finding and Decision." What are the next steps?

A: Following the "Initial Finding," the recipient has 30 days to request that EPB reconsider the case. The request needs to include the reason for reconsideration, whether you would like to appear in person or by phone at the reconsideration, and any new documentation. A reconsideration is the last opportunity to introduce new information or arguments. If a member disagrees with the "Final Finding and Decision," an appeal may be made to the Academy BOD. However, the BOD will not consider new evidence.

Q: I still don't agree with the "Final Decision." How do I appeal to the BOD?

A: A request for an appeal to the BOD must be in writing and sent to the EPB Chair at the Academy office within 30 days of the "Final Decision." The appeal will be heard at the next BOD meeting, provided that all materials are available to the BOD at least two weeks before the meeting date. An appeal to the BOD is for the sole purpose of a second review of the information and arguments presented to EPB. The EPB, as the governing body of the *COE*, has the responsibility to consider and adjudicate cases involving potential breaches of the ethical practice of its members. Members have a responsibility to provide the EPB with all pertinent information. An appeal is not the appropriate time for new information or arguments; the BOD should not be exposed to information or arguments that were not presented to the EPB, which is the decision-making body. Therefore, the appeal is presented in written format, and the information reviewed to be submitted at the appeal shall precede the BOD's receipt of the material.

Q: How does the EPB ensure that the appeal does not contain new information and that the BOD has all the information needed to reach a just decision?

A: To limit the information and arguments at an appeal to the same information and arguments considered by the BOD, the BOD will have access to all the documents reviewed by the EPB. Additionally, the BOD will review the EPB Chair's summary of the member's arguments presented at the reconsideration and the EPB summary of the deliberation of the *COE* as it pertains to the case. The BOD will also be given the member's written summary of arguments from the reconsideration. The member's summary will be submitted to the BOD at least 60 days prior to the appeal. The EPB and legal counsel for the Academy will review the summary to ensure no new information is introduced. If new information is identified, the member will be contacted for clarification. The member will have two weeks to remove the new information or present written arguments to the EPB explaining how the information in question is not new. The EPB and legal counsel for the Academy will determine if the information in question will be included for review by the BOD. If the material remains controversial, from the perspective of the EPB, the President of the Academy will determine whether the information will be allowed. The BOD will have access to the documents at least two weeks prior to an appeal.

Q: Will the BOD know my identity during the appeal?

A: No. All submissions to the BOD will be de-identified so that the member remains anonymous.

Q: How are the decisions of the EPB reported to the general membership?

A: Circumstances of both cases resulting in discipline and those cases closed without a finding of a violation may be reported in *Audiology Today* and on the Academy Web site (http://www.audiology.org/). Findings are published with the intent of educating Academy members in the area of ethics. When cases are published, personal identifying information is not disclosed.

Q: Why aren't offenders names published in *Audiology Today*?

A: The Academy's legal counsel has advised the BOD that describing the nature of the case and its penalty is all that is necessary to educate the membership. Publishing the name of the member increases the risk of a libel lawsuit. The alternative, publishing the name of the member who is in violation and the specific Rule that was violated (but not *how* the Rule was violated) was considered; however, the BOD preferred that the circumstances be described, so that other members would gain an understanding of what is, and is not, a violation of the *COE*.

Q: How are EPB members selected? How can I volunteer?

A: Members serve rotating three-year terms, so positions open each year. When there is a vacancy, the EPB asks the BOD for their recommendations, and those individuals are asked to apply; the EPB also considers those who have expressed an interest to an EPB member. If interested in serving on the EPB, send a letter of intent and resume to the Chair of the EPB. The EPB narrows the list of those who are interested and forwards two names for each opening to the BOD. The EPB members are appointed by the BOD.

Chapter 11

Ethical Conflicts and Dilemmas

Ethical Practice Board of the American Academy of Audiology, 2004–2005

If the difference between right and wrong were clear and agreed on by all, we would probably need no judges or ethical practice boards. Unfortunately, that is not the case. Sometimes the answer is clear: we should not copy the answers from our classmate's exam; we should not accept cash for referring a patient or recommending a specific hearing aid. In the examples below, we have tried to present scenarios that are not always quite as obvious. In some cases the correct behavior seems easily discernible; in others it is not—thus, the dilemmas. In Chapter 3 you learned the basic approach to addressing ethical conflicts and dilemmas. The cases below are provided so that you can deliberate alone or with your colleagues to see if you can reach a consensus. In most of these cases there is no absolutely correct or absolutely incorrect decision. Sometimes we have provided possible courses of action. Remember also that sometimes it is not whether the behavior is legally or morally wrong but whether it is *perceived* to be so (as in Caesar's wife's behavior[1]). Most of the cases below are based on real data—but they were not necessarily referred to the Ethical Practice Board (EPB) of the American Academy of Audiology (Academy).

"COMMIT TO SIX AND THE GOODIES ARE FREE"

A hospital-based audiology practice is affiliated with a cochlear implant center, and about 12–18 patients per year are implanted. The center has successfully used the Brand X implant device for years. The sales representative announces a new incentive program: commit to purchasing six cochlear implants within the next 12 months and the company will give you a free "loaner" cochlear implant processor. The processor is of use only to patients, has no direct benefit to the clinic, and could not be sold separately. The clinic has no ability to purchase a loaner for patients. Since a patient with a broken processor is deaf until the unit is repaired, it would benefit patients to have the extra processor on hand. This deal is in direct conflict with the Academy's *Ethical Practice Guidelines on Financial Incentives from Hearing*

Instrument Manufacturers (Appendix 1), which parallel the conflict of interest guidelines of the AMA/Pharma (Pharmaceutical Research and Manufacturers of America) and rule out obtaining any "perks" that reward for past purchases or commit the audiologist to future purchases, even when he or she will not benefit financially and patients will be helped. What would you do?

EXCLUSIVE REFERRALS?

The local hospital in this moderate size town has served as the primary referral site for private practitioners to send their patients requiring electrophysiologic testing and balance assessment. Jane Steadyman, an audiologist at the hospital, has a reputation for excellence in both estimating hearing sensitivity using auditory brainstem response testing (ABR), and evaluating and managing patients with balance problems. Private practitioners have for many years sent patients needing this testing to Jane. Not only has this arrangement allowed patients to have expert testing and treatment, but the private practice audiologists have not had to invest in the expensive equipment needed to manage these patients. At the state Academy affiliates meeting, Jane tells her colleagues the bad news: The hospital was purchased by another corporation, and the actuaries are closing the audiology program. Jane would like to open her own practice and is willing to limit the practice to electrophysiology and balance work. She will conduct routine hearing testing but will not dispense hearing aids, providing the patients who need amplification a list of referral sources in the community. But to do this, she needs one concession from her colleagues. They must all promise that they will refer at least the same number of patients as they had previously. For the business to succeed, Jane will actually need a little more business than they had sent her before. Is it appropriate for Jane to ask? Is it appropriate for her colleagues to agree to her request?

IMPAIRED COLLEAGUE

A colleague appears to have a problem with alcohol. You are increasingly suspicious that he is starting to drink around 3:30 in the afternoon. You confront him, and he admits that he is having problems. You tell him you are obliged to report him. He begs you to wait. He says he will enter treatment and that, in fact, he has been to Alcoholics Anonymous a time or two but keeps falling off the wagon: "Give me six months. I'll be clean by then." Should you report him, or should you give him the chance he requests? Would your response be different if he were your employer?

ROUTINE TESTING FOR GENETIC DEFECT

It is the year 2015, and the reports we heard of the possibility of detecting Connexin 26 carriers have come to pass (Kenneson and Boyle, 2004). We can not only give parents information on whether they might be carriers so they can be screened for this defect prior to making parenting decisions, but the day has come when the parents can test the fetus to determine if it actually has both recessive genes for the defect. If so, the baby will have a hearing loss, which might be mild to moderate or could be profound. Is it acceptable for society to make this testing available? Many Deaf individuals fear the loss of their culture and disdain the concept that their difference (being Deaf) is a disability—let alone the reason to abort a child. If society allows selective abortion of fetuses with a genetic defect for hearing loss, can we allow selective abortion for hearing babies? There has already been a case in which two Deaf individuals wanted genetic information to assure that the child they brought into the world was Deaf. What will our responsibility be as audiologists if the above scenario does come to pass?

SECOND OPINION

A family approaches you for a second opinion on the diagnosis of hearing impairment in their child. You concur with the previous diagnosis and validate the audiogram. The parents mention the aid recommended. You believe it is an acceptable choice, although not the brand you would have selected. However, you find that the aid recommended by the audiologist who first saw the child is significantly more expensive than your charge for dispensing either that brand or the brand you prefer. This difference is about $1200. You could (a) Tell the parents that you concur that their child has a hearing loss and needs amplification such as that previously recommended, and refer them back to the original audiologist; (b) Do as in option "a" and then contact the referring audiologist and tell him or her you think the price is too high; (c) Tell the parents your price for dispensing the same aid—as well as your preference for another brand. Which option would you choose?

TEEN REBELLION

A severely hearing-impaired patient of yours is now reaching 16. Had he been identified today, he would be considered a candidate for a cochlear implant, but he is a product of past traditions that said his level of benefit from his hearing aids was too great to warrant implantation. He has found hearing aids increasingly of no value. He signs in the classroom and increasingly has a Deaf identity. He has no interest in cochlear implants and now reports that he has lost his hearing aids. He admits in front of his parents that he has no interest in wearing hearing aids. His parents insist that he own them, and they occasionally force him to wear them, for instance, at family reunions. The child is on Medicaid, so the state will pay for the hearing aids. You know that all state Medicaid programs are under severe budget restrictions and, in fact, that your state has ceased to provide hearing aids for anyone over the age of 18 because of financial limitations. The parents want you to order a pair of aids, as the child is entitled to them. What will you tell the child, the parents, and Medicaid?

COMPETENCY AND SKILLS

A large hospital purchased ABR equipment for use in the audiology/ENT department. Following a learning period, two audiologists began testing patients on a regular basis. They test both children and adults. The more skilled audiologist then leaves the position, leaving the less skilled audiologist to hire a replacement. The replacement audiologist has had some experience with ABR, but not in a hospital setting. Upon taking the job, four to five ABRs per week are completed by this new audiologist. In most of the cases, the audiologist concludes that there is enough difference in the waveforms of most patients that a retrocochlear problem cannot be ruled out, and states this on the ABR report. Of course, the report prompts the referring physician to order imaging studies. Analysis of the patients seen by the audiology section reveals that approximately 70 percent of the patients seen for ABR were also seen for imaging following the ABR. Does this circumstance hint at inadequacy on the part of the audiology ABR team? Is this non-rule-out rate consistent with the literature concerning ABR and space-occupying lesions? Should the audiologists have taken different action? Was the training of either or both audiologists sufficient to do these studies? Should they consider additional training; should they abandon the use of ABR evaluations; or should they seek to have a more experienced audiologist hired?

THE INCOMPETENT (?) AUDIOLOGIST AND OTOLARYNGOLOGIST

The audiologist from the school system contacted you, a private practitioner, to dispense amplification to a five-year-old male with a 35–45 dB sensorineural hearing loss. He was previously seen by an ear, nose, and throat (ENT) physician and another audiologist in another office. They made no referral for amplification but suggested a six-month recheck to assess his progress. This is the third child you have fitted in a six-month period for amplification of a mild-to-moderate (or greater) sensorineural hearing loss that was not appropriately treated by the initial ENT/audiology practice; there may be more similar cases that have not come to your attention. You have dispensed hearing aids to the three children identified. All have done remarkably well. Should you (a) Discuss your concern with the otolaryngologist and the audiologist? (b) Report the physician to the state medical board and the audiologist to the state audiology licensure board? (c) Advise the parent to return to the otolaryngologist and the audiologist to discuss their concerns? (d) Write a report to the child's primary care physician to advise them of the difference of opinion so they are aware of that difference and are able to avoid future referrals to these less than stellar professionals? (e) Contact the American Academy of Otolaryngology—Head and Neck Surgery and the American Academy of Audiology to report a violation of the professional codes of ethics? Or should you do all of the above or none of the above?

Ethics in Audiology

A HURTING CHILD

A six-year-old girl who has been treated off and on for three years for recurring ear infections returns to the audiology clinic with her mother for a reevaluation. You note that the child appears quiet and withdrawn and not as outgoing as she had been on previous appointments. In addition, when you move to her right ear to perform tympanometry, she flinches away from you when you attempt to put the probe into her canal, and you notice severe bruising around her ear and neck. You ask her if she remembers getting hurt, and she is evasive initially, but after looking at her mother for a moment, the child states that she fell off her bike. You proceed, very gently, with the testing and then explain the results to the mother. As the tympanogram results indicate another possible ear infection, you recommend that the mother take the child to the pediatrician for immediate follow-up. The mother appears eager to leave the office and is noncommittal about the necessary medical follow-up. Your concern is not only for the flat tympanogram, indicative of some form of middle ear pathology, but also for your suspicion as to the possibility of physical abuse based on the physical presentation of the child as well as the behavioral changes. Should you report the suspected abuse? If so, should you contact the pediatrician or go directly to the appropriate local authorities? You know that child abuse can happen in any family. In the majority of child abuse cases, the child and the abuser are related; at the least, they are known to each other. You also know that you do not need the child's permission to contact the local authorities with your suspicions. The following URL will link you to the National Clearinghouse on Child Abuse and Neglect Information's Reporting Child Abuse and Neglect Web page: http://nccanch.acf.hhs.gov/topics/reporting/index.cfm.

A BIG SHOT IN THE CLINIC

As an audiologist in a large metropolitan area, you are used to many different kinds of patients coming to your clinic for evaluation, diagnosis, and treatment of their hearing and balance problems. Frequently, high-profile patients who are seen routinely in the newspaper and on television contact you for an appointment. Although you attempt to maintain proper patient confidentiality and security according to federal HIPAA guidelines, you cannot account for the proper behavior of others. So, on Monday, "The Patient" comes into your clinic for an evaluation for hearing problems he has been experiencing, and you do all you can to secure the privacy of the patient. You escort the patient to the test area, administer all tests needed, counsel the patient on the diagnosis and treatment options, and schedule a follow-up visit. As the patient leaves the clinic and you get ready to take your next patient in for testing, you overhear a colleague of yours on the telephone in his office talking (gossiping) with someone about The Patient. What is your responsibility? Should you reprimand your colleague? Should you report this breach of confidentiality to your supervisor or the clinic director? If this occurred in your private practice and an audiologist who worked for you made the telephone call, what would your responsibility be? Must you report this violation to the Academy EPB?

DEGREES AND TITLES

Your coworker and you have master's degrees in audiology from regionally accredited institutions. Your university granted you an "M.A." Your coworker was granted a degree from a university that grants an "M.Au.D." to their master's students. The university started granting this designator prior to any university granting the "Au.D." You are considering using the same "M.Au.D." after your name to help identify yourself as a master's degreed audiologist. Is this appropriate?

CONSEQUENCES OF COPYRIGHT VIOLATION

An economically disadvantaged student receives the following offer from her friend: "I'll buy the *Ethics in Audiology* book and let you copy it." Is this legal? Would the offer be made if the copyright violation were likely to be discovered? Is it ethical? What are potential unintended consequences if the Academy does not receive income from the various products it produces?

REPORTING RESEARCH

In your private practice you have recognized a pattern of hearing aid success with a particular type (not necessarily brand) and fitting strategy. You believe your colleagues would benefit from this information. Should you try to publish the results? If so, is there any type of clearance that you should obtain from the patients before submitting the information? (They will not be identified by name or address.) Can you submit the research report without the study having been approved by an institutional review board?

NOTE

1. Caesar's second wife, Pompeia, was accused of scandalous behavior at the annual Feast of the Great Goddess. Caesar demanded a divorce, although there was uncertainty about whether Pompeia had committed adultery, saying, "Ceasar's wife must be above suspicion."

REFERENCE

Kenneson A, Boyle C. (2004) From epidemiology to clinical practice: the connexin connection. In: Khoury MJ, Little J, Burke W, eds. *Human Genome Epidemiology: A Scientific Foundation for Using Genetic Information to Improve Health and Prevent Disease.* Oxford: Oxford Press. http://www.cdc.gov/genomics/training/books/huge/chap24.htm.

Appendix 1

This document was originally published in *Audiology Today*, May/June 2003 (Vol. 15, No. 3), pp. 19–21.

Ethical Practice Guidelines on Financial Incentives from Hearing Instrument Manufacturers

ETHICAL GUIDELINES

The following general guidelines have been accepted by the Board of Directors of the Academy of Dispensing Audiologists (ADA) and the American Academy of Audiology (AAA):

1. When potential for conflict of interest exists, the interests of the patient must come before those of the audiologist.

Any gifts accepted by the audiologist should primarily benefit the patient and should not be of substantial value. Gifts of minimal value ($100 or less) related to the audiologist's work (pens, earlights, notepads, etc.) are acceptable. Incentives or rewards based upon product purchases must not be accepted. This would include cash, gifts, incentive trips, merchandise, equipment, or credit towards such items. No "strings" should be attached to any accepted gift.

Audiologists should not participate in any industry-sponsored social function that may appear to bias professional judgment or practice. This would include accepting invitations to private convention parties, golf outings or accepting such items as theater tickets. Meals and social functions that are part of a legitimate educational program are acceptable. When social events occur in conjunction with educational meetings, the educational component must be the primary objective with the meal/social function ancillary to it.

2. Commercial interest in any product or service recommended must be disclosed to the patient.

This would include owning stock or serving as a paid consultant and then dispensing that product to a patient.

3. Travel expenses, registration fees, or compensation for time to attend meetings, conferences or seminars should not be accepted directly or indirectly from a manufacturer.

Trips sponsored by a manufacturer that are solely educational may be accepted, provided the cost of the trip is modest and acceptance of the trip does not reward the audiologist for past sales or commit the audiologist to future purchases. Faculty at meetings and consultants who provide service may receive reasonable compensation honoraria, and reimbursement of travel, lodging and meal expenses.

4. Free equipment or discounts for equipment, institutional support, or any form of remuneration from a vendor for research purposes should be fully disclosed and the results of research must be accurately reported.

All materials, presentations, or articles produced as a result of the investigation should also carry a disclosure of the funding source. Investigators should structure research agreements with industry to insure that the results are represented accurately, and presentation of findings is objective.

FREQUENTLY ASKED QUESTIONS

Q. Why are AAA and ADA reviewing gift giving from manufacturers?

A. Gift giving from the hearing health care industry to audiologists has been a customary practice. Gifts serve two functions. First, they remind audiologists of the name of the product made by that company. Second, they help a company establish a relationship with the audiologist. However, if the decisions made by the professional are, or appear to be, influenced by an incentive or reward, or can be viewed as not being made objectively, then a conflict of interest may be present. The professional's belief that he or she is not personally influenced is not sufficient to avoid the appearance of a conflict of interest. Our organizations encourage manufacturer/audiologist interactions that serve to improve patient care. However, it is important that gifts do not have the potential to impact professional judgment.

Q. Why would audiologists want to adhere to these guidelines?

A. Audiologists must be committed to the principles of honesty, integrity, and fairness. The principle of putting patients' interests first is the basis of all healthcare professions. Adhering to these guidelines reflects positively on our profession. All healthcare profession licensure acts set limits on professional behavior. In return for a license, professionals are obliged to adhere to certain standards of conduct and have the obligation to self-regulate. Additionally, adhering to a uniform code of ethical conduct may prevent the audiologist from unintentionally violating federal and state regulations.

Q. If an audiologist accepts gifts, what are the potential legal consequences?

A. Acceptance of gifts may not only be construed as constituting a conflict of interest; it may also be illegal. Federal laws make it a criminal act for an audiologist who provides services to Medicare, TRICARE, Medicaid and VA patients to solicit or receive "any remuneration (including any…rebate) directly or indirectly, overtly or covertly, in case or in kind…in return for purchasing…or ordering any goods or services…" Medicare already indirectly covers hearing aids through some private Medicare HMO plans. The Office of the Inspector General has recently issued guidelines for gift-giving activities for the pharmaceutical industry and physicians that appear directly analogous to the issues covered for audiologists in this guideline.

Q. Are incentive trips, vacation packages, gift certificates, cruises, and credits toward equipment purchases or cash received from manufacturers allowed?

A. No. The acceptance of such gifts, whether related to previous purchases or future purchases, raises the question of whether the audiologist is, in fact, holding the patient's interests paramount. There can be no link between dispensing or referral patterns and gifts.

Q. What is the difference between acceptance of trips, lease arrangements, gifts, or receiving a larger discount level?

A. Establishing any type of savings plan with a specific manufacturer creates the appearance of a conflict of interest. Discount programs, however, are generally protected by the law if they have the potential for benefiting consumers. Discount programs are considered to present ethical issues only if they involve commitments by the audiologist that compromise professional judgment.

Q. Can an audiologist accept a trip to a manufacturing facility for the purpose of training?

A. Obviously, there are times when it is more economical and/or a better educational experience can be provided when audiologists are trained together regionally or at the manufacturer's facility. While it is preferable that audiologists pay their own travel expenses, there are circumstances where it is appropriate to accept tickets and/or hotel accommodations:
- The travel expenses should only be those strictly necessary.
- The conference or training must be the reason for the trip.

- Participation must not be tied to any commitment to manufacturers.
- The expense for a spouse or other travel companion may not be compensated by the manufacturer.

Q. Can an audiologist accept a lunch/dinner invitation from manufacturer's representative in order to learn about a new product?

A. Yes, modest business related meals are acceptable.

Q. What are the ethical considerations regarding attendance at sponsored social events at conventions or training seminars?

A. The following criteria should be considered before attending such events:
- The sponsorship of the event should be disclosed to, and open to, all registrants.
- The event should facilitate discussion among attendees.
- The educational component of the conference should account for a substantial amount of the total time spent at the convention.

Q. May an audiologist or a corporation obtain a loan from a manufacturer in order to purchase equipment and then repay a portion of the loan with every hearing aid purchased?

A. Audiologists are encouraged to obtain financing through recognized lending institutions or the equipment manufacturer to avoid potential conflict of interest. Repayment should include only repayment of the debt plus appropriate interest fees but with no additional considerations or obligations on the part of either party.

Q. May an audiologist "co-op" advertising costs with a manufacturer?

A. If the manufacturer wishes to share the cost of an advertisement that features both the manufacturer's name and the audiologist's name, this is acceptable as long as there are no strings attached.

Q. Is it acceptable for a manufacturer's representative to assist in seeing patients at an 'open house' at the audiologists' clinical facility?

A. Open houses are usually product or manufacturer specific with a manufacturer's representative in attendance. The consumer should be very much aware that the presentation would be focused on the purchase of hearing instruments from the featured manufacturer. However, the audiologist still has the responsibility to utilize the most appropriate instruments. The audiologist should consider the legal and ethical ramifications involved if a non-audiologist participates in the open house.

Q. Is there a potential conflict of interest if an audiologist joins a network or buying group?

A. Businesses and organizations are free to negotiate prices on products either directly with the manufacturer or by using the purchasing power of a buying group.

Q. If an audiologist is hired by a corporation that provides hearing aids or other related devices and is offered stock options, is there a cause for concern regarding conflict of interest?

A. If the stock is in the corporation the audiologist works for, there is no conflict of interest.

Q. Are there conflicts of interest implications for researchers?

A. One of the researcher's responsibilities is to fully disclose the funding of the research, whether it is in the form of direct grants, equipment grants or other forms of compensation such as a consultantship with a sponsor. This allows the consumer of the research to evaluate the potential for conflicts of interest. Additionally, researchers are ethically responsible for ensuring the rigor of the scientific design of the experiment and the accuracy and integrity of the interpretation.

Q. Will a similar document on ethical practice guidelines be written for audiologists involved in research and academia?

A. Yes. A set of guidelines is in development to address conflicts of interest in research.

Q. How will the ethical guidelines be enforced?

A. Given the increased enforcement of anti-kickback, fraud, and abuse laws, audiologists should stay abreast of changes in regulatory landscape, and establish procedures and protocols that will protect them in their employment settings and practices. These guidelines are not meant to address all possible interactions but are an effort to assist the audiologist in cases of ethical dilemmas. At this point, education of our members is our focus. However, any profession that fails to monitor misconduct and enforce its Code of Ethics invites the loss of autonomy and the loss of trust in the profession. When such activities exist, the profession must have appropriate disciplinary procedures in place.

Appendix 2

Ethics in Audiological Research
Yvonne S. Sininger, Ph.D.

Early in 2003 I was asked to chair a task force, Ethics in Audiology Research, for the Ethical Practice Board (EPB) of the American Academy of Audiology (Academy). The charge of the new task force was to evaluate current ethical issues in research and create a report for the EPB and Board of Directors (BOD) of the Academy. The task force members were involved in various types of research, in both hospital and university settings. Between the various members, we had been involved in all levels of research, from animal to human, from electrophysiology to hearing aids; we had collaborated with industry and had funding from a wide variety of agencies. Most important, we had all been subjected to ethical training in research and been involved with institutional review at our various organizations. The task force was prepared to discuss issues regarding ethics in clinical research that we felt were relevant to audiologists, and to try to provide guidance to the Academy on needs for dissemination of such information.

The areas of importance that we chose to address included principles of protection of human subjects, ethical practice in authorship of publications and presentations, adequacy of research design and protection of data, and finally, potential conflict of interest in product-oriented outcomes research. These were issues that we as researchers addressed every day, but we felt that the Academy membership may not be aware of these concerns. The task force provided specific recommendations to the EPB. The recommendations, along with supporting rationale, were forwarded to the Academy BOD. Subsequent to their approval, the recommendations were disseminated to the relevant committees. As a result of this report, the *Code of Ethics* was modified to more explicitly address research ethics; therefore, the references to the *Code of Ethics* in the report apply to the version in effect in 2003. The task force report follows.

This document was originally published in *Audiology Today*, Nov./Dec. 2003 (Vol. 15, No. 6), pp. 14–17.

Guidelines for Ethical Practice in Research for Audiologists

Task Force on Ethics in Audiology Research
Yvonne Sininger, Chair; Roger Marsh; Brian Walden; Laura Ann Wilber

PROTECTION OF HUMAN SUBJECTS

The explosion of biomedical and behavioral research in the last half of the twentieth century has brought about scrutiny of the ethical principles by which investigators should be guided. The Belmont Report of the National Commission for the Protection of Human Subjects of Biomedical and Behavioral Research, released in 1979, describes three basic ethical principles that should guide research. These are 1) *Respect for Persons* (the choices of autonomous persons are to be respected and those with diminished autonomy should be protected); 2) *Beneficence* (an obligation to secure the well being of persons by not harming them and by maximizing the benefit-to-risk ratio); and 3) *Justice* (an equality in the sharing of risk and benefits). The Belmont Report is noteworthy for its breadth, addressing many concerns that trouble investigators and others today. Many academic institutions cite it as the ethical standard to be applied in approving research under their jurisdiction. Internationally, the Declaration of Helsinki is often the standard by which human-subjects research is judged, although it is specific to medical as opposed to behavioral, research.

In 2000, the Office for Human Research Protection (OHRP) was established under the Department of Health and Human Services. The OHRP oversees and regulates all aspects of federally funded human research in the U.S. Research institutions involved in federally funded research must have oversight by a local Institutional Review Board (IRB) and must have written "Assurance of Compliance" approved by OHRP. Other institutions can obtain "federal-wide" assurance of compliance by promising to follow general rules and guidelines. In either case the research must comply with the Common Rule, the regulation that governs nearly all federally funded research. Some research, whether or not conducted at institutions that receive Federal support, is subject to other regulations. Many studies of diagnostic and prosthetic devices are subject to FDA regulations, which are very similar to the Common Rule. The Privacy Rule, a HIPAA regulation, governs the use of health information in research.

Individuals with clinical expertise and experience often perform research in audiology. It is incumbent on everyone involved in research to insure that they are appropriately trained to conduct the research in which they are involved. If they have not had formal research training, it is their responsibility to collaborate with other trained researchers to insure compliance with all ethical and legal guidelines as well as use good research design and analysis. Investigators cannot always rely exclusively on their IRB for guidance; the investigator has the obligation to insure the ethical and legal conduct of the study. IRBs vary widely in the expertise and training of their members, so that IRB approval may not be sufficient assurance that the study conforms to ethical and legal standards. Finally, some research is not subject to Federal regulation, and the investigator must assume sole responsibility to assure that it is conducted with proper regard to accepted ethical standards.

Audiologists may be involved in activities that are not generally regarded as research but which involve many of the same ethical concerns. Academy members involved in these activities may not even appreciate the need to consider ethical issues. One example is the published case report. Such reports may not be considered research by some, but these reports have the potential to expose patients' identities, for example if a case report features unusual and/or easily recognized situations. Ethical concerns may arise when a clinician acquires familiarity with a new diagnostic test or device by using it with patients who have little prospect of benefit, or when tests are administered because the clinician anticipates their value in a future research presentation or publication, rather than from clinical necessity.

Existing provisions of the *Code of Ethics* of the Academy are relevant to many of these issues. *Principle 1* ("..honesty and compassion...respect") states important principles underlying human research. *Principle 3* (confidentiality) is clearly relevant. *Principle 4* ("Members shall provide only services...in the best interest") addresses unnecessary services, such as tests that are not clinically indicated. However, this principle raises the potential for ethical dilemmas among clinical researchers who, in controlled clinical trials, may not act solely in the best interest of the patient. In these cases, the appropriate consent process is necessary to clarify the risk/benefit ratio to the prospective subject. *Principle 5* ("Members shall provide accurate information....") embodies the requirement of informed consent, and is the only principle that explicitly addresses research. *Principle 8* already addresses the need to comply with government regulation ("Rule 8b: Individuals shall not engage in...illegal conduct"). However, the Code quite naturally focuses on the conduct of members in providing professional services. It is nearly silent as to the special obligations of members engaging in human-subjects research.

AUTHORSHIP IN PUBLICATION AND PRESENTATION OF RESEARCH

Rapid publication of scientific findings as well as peer review of such manuscripts for quality was born from a need to properly acknowledge credit for scientific discoveries as well as controlling publication quality. Scientists establish credit for their scientific discoveries by publishing them in peer-reviewed journals. The order of authorship carries great importance for establishing relative contributions to the work, including the original ideas. Because there are no hard, fast rules that govern authorship assignment (although guidelines have been published by a variety of sources), the current system is open to abuse.

Research audiologists and hearing scientists often work in groups. For that reason, they must develop rules for deciding how to determine the relative contribution and value of each contributor when assigning authorship to publication and presentation of research. Persons who participate in audiologic research should be appropriately recognized with authorship. Similarly, authorship should not be given to a person who has made little or no contribution to the work, and/or without their consent. In the latter instance, the scientist appears to endorse research about which s/he may have little involvement or knowledge. In other instances, persons may attempt to use their position of authority (department head, section chief, etc.) to secure authorship without actually contributing to the research in a substantial way.

Ethical problems may arise when potential conflicts of interest are not fully disclosed by an author of a research article or presentation. When private companies fund research, such sponsorship must be clearly acknowledged in publications and presentation of the data. Such disclosure should contain details on degree and type of support for specific projects, or general laboratory support.

Authorship and inventorship is highly valued and can be the basis for professional advancement or continued funding of research. Employment, promotion and tenure at universities depend upon an active record of publications and patents. Publications and patents are the signs of achievement for any scientist. Such value in authorship and inventorship can lead to significant abuse. Guidelines on determination of authorship vary somewhat across fields and across institutions or laboratories. Generally the first author is given highest credit and others follow in order. In some groups, the research group leader is last author. In some laboratories, the supervisor's name never appears in the title list and in others it always appears.

According to the International Committee of Medical Journal Editors, authorship should be based on the following criteria: 1) Substantial contribution to conception and design of the research, and/or analysis and interpretation of data and 2) drafting the article or revising its critically important intellectual content and 3) final approval of the version to be published. Accordingly, gift or unwanted authorship is discouraged.

ADEQUACY OF RESEARCH DESIGN AND PROTECTION OF DATA

It is the responsibility of those involved in clinical research to insure that sound experimental design is used and to seek additional training, assistance or collaboration if necessary and appropriate. If a study fails to achieve its objectives because of inadequate sample size, poorly matched controls, or other deficiencies, the potential benefits of the study and the advancement of knowledge are reduced. This, in turn, increases the risk to benefit ratio thus compromising the human subjects in the study. In the worst case, inaccurate conclusions are drawn from poorly designed studies leading to misinformation to clinicians and inconvenience or even harm to patients.

Regardless of outward intent, bias can be reflected in conclusions drawn from research. Given the nature and purpose of the enterprise, science should be objective. The primary interest of scientists should be the discovery of truth. However, when conflicts of interest exist, scientists can be susceptible to protecting their self-interests at the expense of objective science. Outcomes may be assumed prior to the collection and analysis of data. The actual collection and analysis, not to mention the written conclusions, can be biased toward outcomes that are favorable to the author's point of view. Even without intent to manipulate conclusions, poor research methodology can lead to incorrect conclusions. The implications of biased or poor science on a healthcare profession go beyond the introduction of misinformation into the body of knowledge that comprises a discipline. Rather, it can result in the eventual clinical mismanagement of the patients whom the profession exists to serve.

Adhering to established standards when conducting and presenting research is part of the ethics of science. Adherence to the scientific method does not guarantee that research will be error free. Yet, mistakes can be minimized when scientists carefully follow basic scientific principles and accepted practice.

- *Replication.* One important principle of science is to report methodology in a way sufficient to allow for a body of research to be replicated. It is imperative that results hold up to scrutiny at the level of replication, if the truth is to be determined and believed. Scientists must include explicit detail on research design and analysis methodology. In this way other scientists will be able to prove or disprove conclusions by being able to repeat experiments.

- *Standard design, methods and analysis.* Research must be designed, executed, and analyzed to minimize bias or incorrect results. When comparing two clinical techniques, for example, it would be important for the scientist to ensure that each technique is optimized for the particular clinical application before the comparison is made. To do otherwise biases the comparison. Double–blind, cross-over, and other designs that help to eliminate bias, should be employed whenever possible. Data analyses must follow accepted statistical standards and practices. Appropriate education in statistics, as well as consultation with statisticians when appropriate, is recommended for all researchers.

- *Accurate data collection and analysis.* During data collection, meticulous record keeping is essential. Carefully controlled experimental methodology, including documentation and data management following established techniques, is required for the conduct of research. These procedures serve to insure that the scientific and clinical communities will accept the research findings.

CONFLICT OF INTEREST IN PRODUCT-ORIENTED
OUTCOMES RESEARCH

Accurate research aimed at documenting the efficacy of hearing aids, other auditory prosthetics, and diagnostic tests and equipment is essential to the practice of audiology. Most of the research evaluating these products is generated internally by the manufacturers, or is sponsored by manufacturers. Manufacturers often employ audiologists and auditory scientists to evaluate and promote their products. In other instances, product-oriented research is sponsored by industry to be carried out in audiology clinics in a variety of settings. The American Academy of Audiology acknowledges the value of close collaboration between industry, audiologists and auditory scientists in the development and evaluation of new technology for our profession. In fact, such collaboration is felt to be indispensable. However, the employment and sponsorship of Academy members by manufacturers to conduct and report product-oriented outcomes research creates the potential for conflict of interest.

Audiology evolved from primarily an academic discipline, largely centered in educational institutions, into a healthcare profession that focuses on the delivery of clinical services to patients with auditory and balance disorders. Paralleling this evolution has been a change in where, by whom, and why product-oriented outcomes research is conducted. During the early years when audiology was largely an academic discipline, independent faculty scientists with limited or no industry involvement conducted such research primarily in university settings. Gradually, however, responsibility for conducting product efficacy clinical studies has shifted either to the manufacturers of these products, or to independent researchers whose work may be sponsored by those manufacturers.

Although this evolution had been taking place for many years, it received substantial impetus from actions by the federal government in the early 1990's. Primarily in response to consumer complaints that advertising claims of some hearing aid manufacturers were misleading (especially with regard to speech understanding in noise), the Federal Trade Commission (FTC) and the Food and Drug Administration (FDA) charged several major manufacturers with making misleading and/or unsubstantiated claims in advertising about their products. The eventual outcome of these actions was an FDA requirement that hearing aid manufacturers substantiate and obtain pre-market approval of benefit claims in advertising. In order to obtain FDA approval, benefit claims must be substantiated by clinical studies, a portion of which had to be conducted by independent researchers. The result was that hearing aid manufacturers were obligated to conduct efficacy studies of their products within their companies and to support research studies in independent laboratories. As a result, the number of audiologists/clinical researchers employed by manufacturers increased, and several researchers in independent laboratories became engaged in manufacturer-sponsored product efficacy studies.

Within a few years after issuing their ruling requiring hearing aid manufacturers to obtain pre-market approval of benefit claims, the FDA rescinded it. Many Academy members continue to be employed by manufacturers and are involved in conducting and reporting clinical studies of hearing aids and other auditory prostheses. Others receive support for their work through contracts with industry. Additionally, the FDA continues to regulate cochlear implants and middle ear implants, thereby making it virtually certain that audiologists and auditory researchers will continue to conduct efficacy studies of these devices.

A healthcare profession such as audiology, in which the dispensing of products and the use of diagnostic equipment is central to its clinical activities, relies upon outcomes research that accurately assesses the efficacy of those products. Unlike some other professions, such as medicine in which product efficacy studies (pharmaceutical studies) are closely scrutinized by the FDA, studies of hearing healthcare products (i.e., conventional hearing aids and most diagnostic equipment) may receive little government scrutiny. Without efficacy studies that are objective, reliable and carefully executed, audiologists cannot determine which products are best suited to the needs of their patients. The involvement of manufacturers in conducting, reporting, and funding of studies to evaluate their products creates the potential for conflict of interest:

- *Audiologists and Auditory Scientists Employed by Manufacturers.* It is normal and expected that employees will be loyal to their employer. The financial success and security of audiologists and auditory scientists employed by manufacturers is at least partially dependent upon the success of those companies in marketing their products. Hence, it is only reasonable to expect that persons employed by manufacturers will share the commercial goals of their employers and work to achieve those goals. However, as healthcare professionals, audiologists and auditory scientists also have a responsibility always to work toward the best interests of hearing-impaired consumers. It is possible that the commercial interests of manufacturers and the larger professional responsibilities of audiologists and auditory scientists employed by manufacturers may, at times, be conflicting. Often such conflicts may be quite subtle. Nevertheless, Academy members employed by manufacturers must be aware that conflicts in loyalty and responsibility can arise. The potential for conflict of interest needs to be acknowledged. Despite their loyalty and responsibility to employers, it is unethical for Academy members to use poor research designs in clinical studies for the purpose of showing benefit of a particular product, to misrepresent the results of clinical studies of product efficacy, or to misinform/mislead fellow Academy members and/or consumers of the benefits of a particular product.

- *Audiologists and Auditory Scientists Whose Work Is Sponsored by Manufacturers.* Although the potential for conflict of interest among Academy members who are employed directly by product manufacturers may be more obvious, audiologists and auditory scientists whose work is sponsored by manufacturers also are susceptible. The increased sponsorship of product efficacy studies in independent laboratories by manufacturers over the past 10-15 years has involved many Academy members located in academic and/or research settings. Coupled with the generally diminishing availability of intramural funds at these institutions and extramural funding from government agencies, the laboratories of many Academy scientists have become dependent to a greater or lesser extent on funding from manufacturers. With this dependence comes the potential for conflict of interest. Naturally, manufacturers are happy when clinical studies support the efficacy of their products and disappointed when the opposite occurs. Just as audiologists and auditory scientists who are employed directly by manufacturers quite naturally want to please their employers, similarly persons whose laboratories are dependent upon manufacturer funding want to please their sponsors. Again, the potential for conflict of interest needs to be acknowledged. Notwithstanding any financial dependence on manufacturers, it is unethical for Academy members who conduct product efficacy studies to use poor research designs in clinical studies for the purpose of showing benefit of a particular product, to misrepresent the results of clinical studies of product efficacy, or to misinform/mislead fellow Academy members and/or consumers of the benefits of a particular product.

The appearance of a conflict of interest may serve to discredit the work of Academy scientists, if such conflicts are not acknowledged and if appropriate safeguards are not taken to insure the integrity of the research. Clearly, it is in the best interest of hearing-impaired consumers whom we serve that Academy members be engaged in product efficacy studies, both as employees of manufacturers and in contractual relationships with industry. It is in the best interests of the Academy and its members, therefore, to implement safeguards to minimize conflicts of interest among audiologists and auditory scientists employed by manufacturers or whose work is sponsored by manufacturers.

SUGGESTED READINGS

Brody, B.A. (1998) *The Ethics of Biomedical Research.* Oxford University Press.

Sieber, J.E. (1992) Planning Ethically Responsible Research. Newbury Park: Sage Publications.

Committee on Science, Engineering and Public Policy, of the National Academy of Sciences, National Academy of Engineering, and Institute of Medicine. *On Being a Scientist: Responsible Conduct in Research.* National Academy Press: Washington DC, 1995.

Faden, R.R. et al.: *Final Report of the Advisory Committee on Human Radiation Experiments.* US Government Printing Office (Stock #061-000-00-848-9). Washington, DC, 1995. In addition to being a thorough and candid history of the radiation experiments, this is an excellent resource on the history of human research ethics and regulation. Also available at tis.eh.doe.gov/ ohre/roadmap/achre/report.html

USEFUL WEB SITES

http://www.fda.gov/oc/ohrt/irbs/default.htm
   "U.S. Food and Drug Administration Information Sheets: Guidance for Institutional Review Boards and Clinical Investigators." Useful guidance documents, plus links to regulations and other documents. Many are of interest to investigators in clinical research, as well as to IRBs and manufacturers, including the following:
   "Emergency Use of Unapproved Medical Devices "
   " 'Off-Label' and Investigational Use of Marketed Drugs, Biologics and Medical Devices"
   "Guidance on Significant and Nonsignificant Risk Devices"

ohrp.osophs.dhhs.gov/index.html
   Office for Human Research Protections. Links to the Belmont Report, the Common Rule (45 CFR 46), as well as educational and guidance documents.

http://www.wma.net/e/policy/17-c_e.html
   "The Declaration of Helsinki of the World Medical Association." This is the most recent version, which has several substantial differences from earlier versions.

http://www.aamc.org/members/coitf
   Protecting Subjects, Preserving Trust, Promoting Progress—Policy and Guidelines for the Oversight of Individual Financial Interests in Human Subjects Research. Task Force on Financial Conflicts of Interest in Clinical Research, Association of American Medical Colleges, December 2000.

Glossary

Ethics 101
Jane M. Kukula, Au.D.

Adjudicate: The act of coming to a decision; to act as judge; to pass judgment.

Altruism: Unselfishness; selflessness; putting others' needs above one's own; looking to others' welfare first.

Appearance: An external suggestion; outward impression or expression.

Autonomous: Self-directing; independent; having the freedom to choose one's own direction, including commitment to right behavior.

Axiomatic: Goes without saying; apparent; obvious; that which is known and generally accepted by others.

Beneficence: To do what is good and right; to perform acts of kindness and charity.

Benevolent: Oriented toward doing good; predisposed to performing acts of kindness and to doing good.

Breach (noun): A violation of the law, an agreement, or an obligation.
(verb): To sever a contract or trust; to break one's commitment.

Casuistry:[1] Ethical decision making made by applying ethical principles or by reviewing cases that have been previously deliberated.

Coerce: To entice another to do one's will; to dominate another's will, to persuade one to choose against his or her will.

Confidence: A belief in another; to place one's trust in another, often in a relationship in which one individual has greater knowledge or authority and the other relies on that knowledge or authority.

Conflict of interest: When the personal interests and the professional duties of a person are at odds; when the potential for personal gain is in conflict with professional decision making; a result of incentives such as cash or trips that entice or create the appearance of enticing professionals to act in their own personal interest.

Deontologic: Having to do with an agreed-upon set of ethics or rules, or with universal rules of right and wrong.

Dilemma: Facing a choice in which one is forced to choose between equally unsatisfactory alternatives; when the correct choice between right and wrong is not apparent.

Discipline (verb): to regulate, to correct, or to punish.

Duty: Behavior that is compulsory; behavior and actions that are required of one's position; professional responsibilities and obligations.

Duty-based ethics: Moral behavior rising out of one's professional responsibilities and obligations, including legal duties.

Ethical: Behavior consistent with accepted professional and moral conduct.

Ethics: The morals and values guiding right and wrong actions within a profession; moral principles; principles or values of a profession.

Fidelity: Loyalty; faithfulness; the devotion to a person, a principle, or an obligation.

Fiduciary: Relating to or involving a confidence or trust; held or founded in trust or confidence.

Fraud: Intentional misrepresentation of the truth in an attempt to influence another to relinquish an item of value. Deliberate distortion of information to achieve personal gain.

Incentive: An item of value offered to influence one's actions; often a gift, cash, or promise of reward in exchange for an action such as purchase of a specific product.

Integrity: Adherence to moral values; personal and professional honesty and truthfulness.

Just: That which is fair, correct, moral, or good.

Justice: Acting with fairness and impartiality; decision making based on what is right and wrong; right or correct behavior.

Litigate: To pursue legal action; to bring about court action.

Malfeasance: Wrongdoing or misconduct; bad behavior.

Misrepresent: To intentionally lie in order to trick or deceive; to purposefully distort the truth or facts.

Moral: Behavior that complies to standards of right and wrong; performing good and just acts; doing that which is honorable and proper.

Negligence: Not providing the normal acceptable standard of care; carelessness and laxity in service delivery.

Nonmaleficience: To do no harm in the delivery of services; not being harmful.

Ought: A moral duty; an ethic one must uphold; an obligatory right act.

Reprimand: A form of discipline used to shape ethical or legal behavior; a chastisement; usually a written notice.

Revocation: Cancellation or rescindment, as of a membership or license.

Right: Correct or true; doing that which is just, good, or proper; an ideal of good or appropriate behavior.

Sanction: Discipline or chastisement used to encourage moral or legal behavior.

Self-interest: Placing one's own welfare above that of others; prioritizing one's own interests over those of others.

Statute: A law; a decree, order, or ruling passed by the legislature.

Suspension: Postponement or delay, as of membership and member benefits.

Teleologic: Being directed in a purposeful manner by an intrinsic set of rules; in nature's design.

Trust: A belief in another to act in a certain manner; to have faith in another's ability or truthfulness; a reliance on another to act on your behalf.

Utilitarian ethics: Ethical decisions based on what will do the least harm to involved parties; the rightness of an action is determined by its outcome.

Veracity: Commitment to truthfulness or authenticity; acceptance and dedication to truth.

Violation: The breach of a law or rule; an infraction.

Virtue: Goodness; behaving in a right or true manner; achieving moral excellence.

Virtue-based ethics: Ethics that is founded in virtues, is altruistic, and requires dedication.

NOTE

1. For those versed in the International Phonetic Alphabet, we offer the pronunciation "kæʒ´ u ɪ stri."

REFERENCES CONSULTED

Beauchamp TL, Childress JF. (1994) *Principles of Biomedical Ethics.* 4th ed. New York: Oxford University Press.

Webster's New Collegiate Dictionary. (1981) Springfield, MA: G. and C. Merriam.

Index

Ethics in Audiology